I SEE,
SAID THE BLIND MAN

Art Seamans

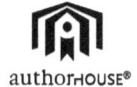

authorHOUSE®

AuthorHouse™
1663 Liberty Drive
Bloomington, IN 47403
www.authorhouse.com
Phone: 1-800-839-8640

First published by AuthorHouse   4/27/2010

ISBN: 978-1-4490-9838-4 (e)
ISBN: 978-1-4490-9837-7 (sc)

Library of Congress Control Number: 2010903184

Printed in the United States of America
Bloomington, Indiana

This book is printed on acid-free paper.

CONTENTS

Acknowledgements

I wish to express my appreciation to a number of assistants and helpers who have made this book possible. My assistants include Morgan Cooper, Lindsay Preston, Dominic Tarantino, and April Anderson. I especially wish to thank April Anderson who served as proofreader to the work. Ernie Loos, Dwight Moyer, Ted Hartley, Rachel Mournian, and the Tamarack Writers Group also gave helpful suggestions to the writing of the book. The photograph of the author on the back page was taken by Marcus Emerson, who gave permission for its use.

The cover design was created by Aletha Anderson.

CHAPTER ONE:

Discovering the World of Blindness

Yesterday, when part of my manuscript was being read, Bethany said, "Tell us your story of how you went blind." Like the Ancient Mariner, I decided to recount the events leading to my blindness. Unlike the Mariner, I was asked to tell the story, and unlike the Ancient Mariner, I will tell the story of land exploration rather than of a sea voyage. I certainly was not born blind, in fact I didn't wear glasses until I was thirty years old; and I had been in the Army. Becoming visually handicapped was the farthest thing from my mind. There were very few eye problems in my family. My second cousin had macular degeneration, and my aunt had glaucoma; however, I can still see my grandmother at age 100 with a magnifying glass reading *The National Geographic*. I sailed along happily with my good eyesight; my glasses were not very high powered. And then, in my sixties I started noticing that it was increasingly difficult to drive at night. I was driving on Route 11 in Upstate New York where it intersects the 91. It was 10:00 at night, and the road had been freshly repaved. No lines had been repainted. I had to stop the car and get out to see where the turn-out to the interstate was. Small print became increasingly difficult to read. In our office the copy machine would blow up the print.

Realizing that I was having some problems, I visited my ophthalmologist, who had me tested on a machine that flashed little lights on a surface. Each time I saw a light flash, I was to press a button. When I had finished the test, the operator of the test looked at me and queried, "Did you *drive* here?" When I answered affirmatively, he shook his head. I have to confess that I drove my car long after I should have. When I drove up A Street in Downtown San Diego, I would move my head around to catch the traffic lights. Then one time I turned onto a highway divider thinking it was a cross street. I almost ran over two pedestrians at crosswalks. I shudder to relate this. I wonder if the most dangerous section out of my exploration occurred at its beginning, before I came to terms with my decrease in vision. In trying to analyze my thinking at the time, I guess I was panicking at the thought of losing my driving ability. I wondered how I would get to work, travel to church, and get to the fitness center.

On observing that I was having eye trouble, my colleague Dean Nelson took me to an acupuncturist. I lay on the exam table. Two Chinese acupuncturists came in. They rubbed a metal rod on my ankles and asked me if I was married. They were most displeased when I said that I was single. "Your trouble," they said, "is not just with your eyes. It's with your kidneys. Your eyes and your kidneys or liver are connected." I started thinking of the song, "The ankle bone is connected to the leg bone, and the leg bone is connected to the hip bone." "What you need to do," they pontificated, "is to stop reading anything immediately. Next, come to our office for treatments once a week. We will give you herbal tea and stick you with pins. The price will be 600 dollars a month.

By the way, bring along all past medical records. The price of this visit will be fifty dollars."

I didn't like the idea of not reading. I didn't like the idea of traveling to La Jolla and paying out 600 dollars a month for a treatment, the effectiveness of which I was unsure. I didn't like their unfriendly attitude to both Dean Nelson and myself. I paid the fifty dollars and shook the dust off my feet as I left. Perhaps that same dust came back to blind my eyes. I don't know. Along with other rescue attempts from this land, I turned this one down. I did not trust these guides to lead me out of the land of darkness. Their needles and their rods did not comfort me. My cup did not run over.

Perhaps they were right in ordering me to stop reading immediately. I don't know. How could I stop reading when I'm trying to earn my living teaching? Well, I made it through a batch of freshman composition research papers until I got to the last sentence of the last paper. Then I discovered that I could read no more. The last glimpse of the shore had vanished.

Believe me, I would not wish to live the year that followed again. My assistant at the time proved to be a very absent help in times of trouble. I guess she was taking care of her young son, but she was not around my office. I fell upon the thorns of life; I bled. I really needed to take some kind of attendance in my classes, but since I could not make out faces very distinctly, I relied on whether the chairs were filled or vacant. Alas, the chairs were movable. Sometimes the students just decided to sit next to some new interest in their lives. Sometimes the chairs just had a way of getting out of line. Chairs in a classroom, like strings placed near each other in a drawer, started automatically to move in strange configurations. Perhaps it's the seventh law of dynamics. Taking attendance became an impossible task.

Then, because of my generous heart, too generous for my own good, I would accept papers slid under the door, passed to me on the way to chapel, stuck in my hands in the restroom, or laid on my desk among various other artifacts. Sometimes these papers were on time; sometimes they were late. Sometimes they were signed; sometimes they were unsigned. Sometimes they identified the class to which they belonged; sometimes they did not identify the class. Sometimes the assignments were identified; sometimes they were not. Sometimes excuses were given for their lateness, sometimes not. The one excuse that stands out in my mind is that given by one young lady who stated that she and her roommate heard a sermon on Sunday on the eminent return of Jesus in the clouds. They therefore had to spend the whole week preparing for the event, which would surely take place before the arrival of the new moon. How could one write a theme when the end of the world as we now know it was about to take place? Once I received these papers, I placed them in my attaché case where they shared accommodations with books, paperclips, mail, syllabi, and vitamin pills.

Then there was the grade book. Grade books are designed for little old ladies that are used to fine knitting. Squeezing a grade in between two faint lines with only a millimeter between them was always a challenge. It became an impossible challenge when my eyes dimmed. The grades started to move around just as the chairs had. Daily work got mixed up with theme grades and midterm examination grades.

The ophthalmologist decided that I had age-related macular degeneration, but he sent me to retina specialist. I didn't even know there were such creatures. I think I had just about every test, thanks to Kaiser Permanente, that exists. They injected me with liquid that would flow through the eyes. They gave me an MRI. They asked me to walk a straight line. They asked me which day of the month it was and what county I lived in. The doctor handed me a pencil and asked me to write a sentence. Now, how do you suppose I was able to hold a position teaching English at a college if I couldn't write a sentence? I did as I was told and wrote the following sentence: "I am thankful for specialists like you who work with eye problems." I slid the paper over to him, and as he read it, a smile crept over his face. How many times did they dilate my eyes and peer into them with lights? After one dilation, I returned to my office barely able to see and with tears streaming down my face. When my secretaries and colleagues saw me, they went into a panic mode, thinking that I had become totally blind. One particularly unpleasant examination consisted of placing electrodes on my eyeballs. One time when I was being examined, the attendant said, "You have to leave." I exclaimed, "W-Why do I have to leave? What have I done wrong?" I was quite indignant. She replied, "Everyone has to leave. There is a bomb threat in the building."

Well, the retina specialist came up with a new diagnosis: "I think you have retinitis pigmentosa," he said. I was obviously forced to learn a new vocabulary about eye diseases.

"What is retinitis pigmentosa?" I asked.

He responded, "Your vision will constantly narrow until you go blind. I don't know why you have it, since it is usually associated with young people. Come back and see me next week," he ordered.

The doctor also informed me that I was legally blind. Well, when I reported that news to my relatives, they really sat up and took notice. The word *blind* was like a red flag waved before a bull. My brother especially decided to view this revelation as a tragedy. The news of my altered condition spread throughout the nation. I never had to tell any of my previous acquaintances that I was blind.

Next week I came back. "I wish to see Dr. X," I said. "He told me to come back." The receptionist said, "You can't see him." No explanation was given. Had he taken a dislike to me? Maybe he was dead. Perhaps he was in prison or had gone insane. No explanation was forthcoming.

"What do I do now?" I asked.

"Well," she said, "you can see Dr. Y." Well, actually I liked Dr. Y better than Dr. X., and after he examined my eyes, which had been dilated of course, he looked at my records.

"Hmmmm," he said, "I don't think you have retinitis pigmentosa. I think you have Stargardt's disease."

"What is that?" I asked.

"Well, you see better out of the periphery of the eye than in the center, and you see better at night than during the day." Was I becoming a werewolf? A night creature? "I don't know why you didn't get it when you were younger," he said. "Anyway, one of my patients is a helicopter pilot. He doesn't want people to know he has eye trouble. He therefore asked to only fly at night. By the way, you won't go totally blind."

I left the office proclaiming to the world that I no longer had retinitis pigmentosa. I had Stargardt's disease. In fact, I had Stargardt's disease for several years, until I retired, signed up with a new plan, and saw another retina specialist. "You have," he said, "age-related macular degeneration." Here we go around the mulberry bush. I had returned to my first diagnosis. Well, I have had age-related macular degeneration to this day. "You won't go blind," he assured me. And to this day I have not gone totally blind. How dull to have age-related macular degeneration! Everybody has it. And dear reader, there's a good chance you'll have it too before too long.

There was nothing to do but to begin coping with my altered circumstance. First, I gave up driving. My last driving trip was to Johnny R's on El Cajon Blvd. After eating breakfast, I exited on El Cajon Blvd. only to be met by street cones. I could not figure out whether to drive to the left of them or to the right of them, and vowed that I would never drive again if I could get that car home safely. I have kept my vow and have sold the car. I drive now only in my dreams.

The second adjustment was to perform my grocery shopping. About the time I started to have eye trouble, I ran into Ted Hartley, an old student of mine. He stated that he would be glad to come to my condo once a week to take me grocery shopping and read my mail. I picked up a grocery cart that can be pulled, and in spite of the wild way that the store mixed up its goods on the shelves, Ted managed to find most of the items on my list. I have no way of checking prices and brand names. I asked a clerk where the oleo margarine was, and the young clerk had no idea. He had never heard of oleo or margarine. I grabbed bags of what I thought were crackers and found out later that they were pork rinds. I grabbed for a can of beets and ended up with pig's feet. I briefly left my shopping cart only to grab the wrong cart, whereupon an angry lady accused me of either being a thief or a villain or both. At the check-out counter the clerks asked me if I wished to have help out to my car. If I had driven a car and was walking with a mobility cane, call the police! The clerk handed me a foot long sales slip and fifty dollars that I had requested all in one swift swoop. Holding my mobility cane in one hand, I tried to separate the sales slip from the fifty dollars to stuff them into my pocket. I have been to Starbucks and the clerk returned the sales slip, two dollar bills, one dime, two nickels, and three pennies in one swift swoop. Some of the change clattered to the floor. I considered that change a tip for the janitor. But, I have survived. Slowly, I was discovering the country of the blind, and its ruts, and its pit falls. Slowly too, I was learning to adapt to this new country.

Teaching presented its own challenges, apart from taking attendance. I could no longer look at notes on a lecture I was to give. Instead, everything I was to teach had to be in my head. This inability to read notes while I lectured turned out to be perhaps a positive. It was like riding a bicycle after they take off the training wheels. With no notes to lean on, I was free to express what I knew, relying only on a mental outline to direct my progress through the lecture. When I had no more to say, I led the class into a discussion or let them go. No student ever complained that I dismissed them before the allotted time. What? No student felt cheated that he didn't get the total hour of class time? Alas, no. It is true, however, that I always forgot one or two points that I meant to say. Forever, these students will be without those precious gems of knowledge, or perhaps factoids.

One problem in teaching I have not yet licked: it seems impossible in a class of fifty to link names to faces I can hardly detect. Students never knew what I could see and what I could not see. I don't think that they were able to get away with much, even if they so desired. To my knowledge I was not like one of my old colleagues, Professor Tillotson. In the middle of his lecture, a student rose and exited his classroom. Tillotson thereupon concluded that his lecture had gone on after dismissal time. Instantly, he ended the lecture, apologizing to the students for keeping them overtime, when in actuality the class time was only half over. One student in a Victorian literature class wrote a letter to the college newspaper about a disrespect that was shown to me—a disrespect that I never saw any evidence of. My skin is fairly thin. I think I would have detected any signs of disrespect. It was later found out that she was losing her own eyesight, and she was probably projecting her fears onto my situation.

I believe that my class discipline was always good because I always obeyed rule number one: one person talks at a time, either me or somebody else. How can students listen to the teacher if more that one person is talking at a time? If a student started talking, I stopped talking until the student stopped. I did have another rule: I did not allow the students to sleep during the lecture. Now, it is true that John would lay his head on the table during Victorian class. But, his eyes were open, and he watched me intently. I never made a big deal about being visually handicapped, and the students didn't make a big deal about it either.

Necessity is the mother of invention as they say. The necessity of keeping papers straight led me to ban all papers from my attaché cases, except student work. Any papers that were passed in late, I would not receive until I had my attaché case handy. The learning center at school provided me with a great favor indirectly: to help students who were having trouble with the literary readings, a reader read the selections aloud into a recording machine that transferred the reading into tapes that could be purchased. I was the one that needed the tapes—badly.

After using the mimeograph machine to enlarge the print of text I needed to read, I made the most important discovery in my attempt to cope with my blindness. On my Christmas vacation, I visited my sister and her family in Florida. She mentioned that the local library possessed a machine that would read texts aloud. My nephew drove me to the library, where I discovered the Reading Edge, a machine invented by Kurzweil. Returning to campus, I told my area dean that instead of obtaining a loan from the school for a computer, I needed the Reading Edge. Instead, Dr. Strawn indicated that the advancement office would write a Mr. Anderson of the Xerox company to ask him and his corporation for a gift to the school of this machine. I still possess that machine, and the SARA machine from Freedom Scientific and the KNFB Reader from KNFB Reading Inc. These machines are technology's greatest gift to the blind. Instead of relying only on taped books, I was able to read almost any book among the millions of books that libraries hold. From struggling up inclines, I now found a level path to lead me around the mountains and through ravines.

When I graded student themes, I made my readers note every capitalization and punctuation mark. Sometimes I had them spell out unusual words that appeared. Naturally, I had to have papers read to me for my evaluation. And so I dwindled into a handicapped person. But my love of learning and my love of teaching only grew.

Since I live alone, I had to learn some coping skills around the condominium. Although I never use the oven and rarely use the burners, I decided to use neither, relying on the microwave. I had to find a microwave that was simple to operate. I eschew microwaves with flush buttons and fancy timing mechanisms. Since I can't read the labels on canned foods or pills, I place both in unique locations. Stewed tomatoes I place behind my water filter. Canned peas I place on top of my refrigerator. Canned stews I place in my cabinet over my plates. I discovered a can opener that solved all my problems in getting at the contents of food in cans. It's a little gadget about the shape of a mouse. After placing it on the can, one can press a button and the machine will do the rest, circling the can until the top is open. Items encased in plastic present another problem. Usually there are instructions at how to open these items, but since I can't read these instructions, I jab the package with a knife or scissors. Plastic will not let itself be torn by hands. Opening medicine bottles presents its own challenge. Does one press down and turn, press tabs on the side and turn, or squeeze the top and turn? The blind person sometimes tries all of these strategies with limited success. I had to get rid of my Oreck vacuum cleaner since it pulled up everything on the floor including socks, underwear, nickels, and papers. I have major problems with my telephone numbers and addresses. I purchased five-by-eight note cards. On one side I wrote the name of the person whose address or phone number appears on the other side. Even though I use a wide black marker, I sometimes cannot read my own writing. These cards I place in a small file container. Sometimes when I'm in a hurry, I write down an address or a phone number and fail to write down to whom it belongs. Then I get strange and wonderful phone calls, especially on my answering machine. One time I came home to hear the following message spoken by a woman: "I'm coming to your house at two this afternoon to give you a bath." Many other times I pick up the phone only to find there is no one on the other end of the phone. Every organization you can think of needs money. Perhaps I am insensitive, but I do not feel like giving money to the Shriners in order for them to put on a Christmas party for handicapped children. Do police organizations really solicit donations on the telephone? Then I am invited to respond to a list of questions for a survey. When I hear, "Do you approve of Councilman X's watching pornography on his computer?" I shut down the receiver in disgust. Another great convenience for the blind is the provision to dial 411 and receive phone numbers around the country. Again, technology has come to the rescue of the blind.

I think that even should I go totally blind, I could manage in my small condominium. There is an old gospel song entitled "I Feel Like Traveling On." One option for coping with my blindness would be to crawl into my cocoon of a condominium and vegetate. For work, worship, pleasure, and exercise, I needed to get out of that cocoon. The first step was to find alternate means of transportation. There were only two options: first, to beg my friends for rides, and second, to take the busses and trolleys. Taking the second option involved coping with the city's transit system. I think I had ridden the busses in San Diego a total of two times before I lost my eyesight. Busses seemed to me to be a considerable nuisance in the road. When I was driving behind a bus, the bus would stop periodically. I could either wait for the bus to begin its movement or try to pass the bus. To me, the busses were simply an irritant. My assistant says, "Busses are the most dangerous thing when you are on a bicycle. They pull out without signaling, cut you off on the curb, blow smoke in your face." Car drivers have their own complaints about busses.

After I became visually handicapped, I learned to bless the busses—not curse them. Getting used to bus travel required some learning. My fears beset me. My first fear was: How do I find the bus stop? The second fear came next: Where do I buy a ticket? My third fear followed: How do I let the driver know where I want to get off? The fourth fear appeared last: What kind of schedule do these busses keep? Do they just drive at random? The poet Arthur Hugh Clough wrote, "If hopes were dupes, fears may be liars." The fears were liars. Bus stops are clearly marked. The busses appear on regular frequent schedules, and are usually on time. To let the driver know when you wish to get off, pull the cord that runs along the side of the bus. Tickets may be purchased at the transit store on Broadway or at your local grocery store. A great boon to the blind is that a ticket for the whole month is only seventeen dollars. Furthermore, I found that I need not waste the time twiddling my thumbs on the bus. It is true that it takes longer to get from point A to point B than driving between the two places, but I can give my undivided attention to my Walkman, listening to music or books on tape. I can relax totally, generally in spite of loud fellow travelers. If I sit close to the driver, I can hear him call out most of the stops. Occasionally, in their eagerness to make a buck, the busses not only carry huge advertisements below the windows, but they envelop the whole bus in an advertisement, including the windows. I have a hard enough time seeing where the bus is without peering through a myriad of paint drops that are part of some inane advertisement.

Although I never feared violence traveling on the bus, occasionally people said to me, "Aren't you frightened riding on the bus?" It is true that one time a couple of teenagers were throwing paper wads at each other near my head, but most people keep to themselves. At least they keep their arms and legs to themselves. Alas, often they do not keep their voices to themselves. Sometimes the bus sounds like the Spanish Inquisition. A favorite trick for some riders is to sit on one side of the bus and converse with someone else on the other side of the bus with everybody else in the middle. Then there are those who feel it incumbent upon themselves to entertain the bus driver with a steady stream of trivia. One young man places his bicycle on the front of the bus, and upon entering the bus announced to the entire audience whatever was on his mind, which wasn't much.

As delightful as San Diego usually is, my world is bigger than San Diego. Doctor Johnson proclaimed, "When a man is tired of London, he is tired of life." Although I'm not tired of San Diego, I do not wish to spend the rest of my life confined to its streets. At the foot of Broadway, I can see the Santa Fe Depot, the Greyhound Bus Terminal, and in the distance, Lindbergh Field. At the harbor, there are cruise ships waiting.

Now, from way back I have enjoyed riding by Greyhound bus. I enjoy looking out the window at the countryside. On the airplane, the countryside looks very much like a toy landscape if one can glimpse any of it through the clouds. On the train, one glimpses all the stockyards, broken down factories, and tumbleweed in the countryside. The view from a seat on the Greyhound bus is spectacular. I like the fact that no reservations are really required to ride the bus. However, bus travel has gone downhill over the last several decades. No longer can you check luggage through to your destination. At each transfer point you have to find your own suitcases on the bottom of the bus and drag them to the next bus. In the old days, you could indicate the route you wished to travel. Now the computer rules and blocks out any attempt of the customer or the ticket agent to plan your route. To go from San Diego to Chicago, I do not wish to swing by Denver. To travel from New York City to St. Louis, I do not wish to go through Pennsylvania, the middle of Ohio, and the middle of Indiana.

Then there are the rest stops. In the old days, the bus would travel to some delightful country restaurant and let you freshen up and eat in a nice forty-five-minute frame. Presently the bus driver allows you ten minutes in a convenience store to rush in and find the restroom and then rush to find a hamburger or a candy bar. If this is difficult for a sighted person, it is impossible for a visually handicapped person. The bus driver lets you out with a stern warning that if you aren't back in ten minutes, the bus will leave without you. Finding the restroom at a convenience store and picking out a decent snack challenged me to the very fiber of my being. I've had to resort to asking strangers if they would help me operate the automatic vending machines. I can't see what the machine is displaying, I don't know how much the fee is, and finding where to put the money is beyond my capabilities. On the last trip I grabbed a bag I was sure was mine since they all look alike. Fortunately the true owner ripped it out of my hand.

On my latest cross country trip, the bus, unlike most busses, was a dog. It held too many people to be serviced by one tiny toilet. My knees were pressing the seat in front of me. When a capacious woman sat next to me on the aisle seat, I felt trapped. Only through the courtesy of the bus driver and strangers did I survive that trip across the country with my mobility cane.

In the old days a trip by air was a luxury. Every customer wore dress up clothes. The stewardesses were lovely and eager to cater to every wish. The food was varied and delicious. Boarding the airplane resembled your arrival at a resort. Alas, those days are gone. Passing through the checkpoint resembles the old "rat race" we used to have in basic training. In the "rat race," which is designed as some kind of punishment for a slow response to falling out of the barracks into formation, the sergeant orders you back into the barracks. In three minutes you are to fall out with gas mask, helmet liner, dress uniform, and rifle. If everyone is too slow falling out, he is given another three minutes to rush back into the barracks and fall out with fatigues, backpack, and dress shoes. These little forays may go on for some time until everyone is exhausted and the sergeant is bored with tormenting everybody. Now I understand the safety concerns in boarding an airplane. I don't mind taking off my shoes, my coat, my jacket, and my watch, or emptying out from my pockets a handful of pennies and quarters, or taking off my belt. What I do mind is performing this in two seconds with people pushing behind me and the belt moving in front of me. After being checked through the screening arch, I then have to reassemble myself while people and coats and umbrellas and shoes and purses swirl around me.

Another challenge for a blind person involves moving from one gate to another when a change of planes is called for. Since I can't see the screens, I have to try to grab the ticket agent. In most airports I have given up trying to walk from one gate to another and must wait for a wheelchair. At O'Hare airport the poor attendant pushed me from one terminal to the other, down five quarters and ten elevators before I arrived at the proper gate. Sometimes at the proper gate, the new attendant has not arrived, and I am not sure I have been delivered to the right gate. All in all, however, I get by with the courtesy of strangers who help me find the restroom, identified only by a tiny little sign.

The best way for me to travel is by train—at least sometimes. On the Sky Chief from Los Angeles to Chicago, I can stretch out in the capacious seats, walk to the lounge car, and appear at the dining car without losing my way. I am safe until I arrive at the train terminal. Oh, that the train from Chicago to Syracuse lived up to the Sky Chief's standards. It is sad that train routes have diminished so markedly over the last fifty years. Recently I have found that authorities had cancelled the train across the Southern United States. To get to Florida from San Diego, one has to go by way of Los Angeles, Chicago, and Washington D.C.—a trip that lasts about four days.

Reluctantly I have learned that I can no longer travel solo when it comes to foreign travel. I must either be in a group or be accompanied by a sighted friend. And so, I have diminished into being a kind of Tiresias on the Road, waving my mobility cane and depending on strangers to be my guide through life.

Occasionally I dream that a book is handed to me, and to my surprise I can read it very easily. "Of course I can read," I say to myself. And in the middle of this dream I wake up and for a moment think that perhaps I can read. I quickly discover that what seemed so simple in the dream is impossible in reality. For people with macular degeneration there is no return to a sighted country. But while I cannot outside of the dream world read, I learn that I can survive and indeed survive very well. The country of the blind has many ruts, and a number of mountains and ravines, but none of these has kept me from enjoying the trip.

CHAPTER TWO:

The Caucus Race

People including me love to give advice. Consequently as an obviously half-blind creature, I have received my due share of suggestions.

One rather persistent one was that I attend the Braille Center or the San Diego Center for the Blind. Inertia kept me from going to either. I didn't know exactly where either was or how to get to either. I didn't know what to expect there at either place. I am always busy. One day at church Troy Potter approached me, mobility cane in hand. "I hear you are legally blind," said Troy. "Why don't you try going to the Blind Center? They even provide transportation to and from the center." One day then, I managed to get up enough gumption to walk to El Cajon Blvd. and catch the 15 bus to 59th Street. I asked the bus driver to please tell me when the bus arrived at 59th Street. At certain intervals he would mumble a street name. Fearing that I would miss the street, I asked the man in front of me where we were. A great silence followed. A woman across the isle stated, "We are at 54th Street. I'll tell you when we get to 59th Street." She lived up to her word.

As I rose to approach the front door of the bus, the driver said, "I told you I would announce when we got to 59th Street."

"Yes" I responded, "But you mumble."

As I exited the bus, I looked around for the center. Like Alice chasing the white rabbit down a hole, I knew I was entering a new world, one that would shake up my normal pattern of life, introduce me to new creatures, and present new challenges. After crossing El Cajon Boulevard, I entered a thrift store. "Where is the San Diego Center for the Blind?" I asked the clerk.

"Don't move a blessed inch," she replied. "You are at it. This is the Blind Center."

The chief director of this new world I had fallen into was a mild-mannered, pleasant man named Mark. I suppose he fulfilled the function of the Dodo bird in Alice's dream. He interviewed me next to the Coke machine, assuring me that many benefits unspecified would emerge from following the program of the center for an unspecified time.

That conversation with Mark was the first introduction I had to what I might call the Caucus Race of Alice in Wonderland fame. You will recall that Alice fell asleep while her sister was reading a history book that unfortunately had no pictures. What ensued was somewhat of a nightmare. She followed a white rabbit that strangely was wearing gloves and a top hat. So fascinated was she by this strange sight that she followed the rabbit into the rabbit hole and ended up trapped in a hallway from which all doors were locked. One door interested Alice because of the garden on the other side. The key to this enticing door lay on a stool. Unfortunately the door was much too small for Alice to enter. On a table she saw a sign next to a cupcake saying, "Eat me." Magically she shrank until she was small enough to enter the door, but then she remembered that she had left the key on the stool and could not reach the key. She then saw a sign that said, "Drink me," and grew so large that she could not see her feet. In fact she was worried that her feet had disappeared. After she had wept a while for the loss of her feet, she ate some more of the cupcake to shrink her size. However, then she found herself awash in her own tears along with other animals such as the eaglet and the mouse. At this juncture, the Dodo bird appeared, saying that if they would run in what he called a Caucus Race, they would dry off. After running for a half-hour in this race, everyone, including Alice, did get dry. So the Caucus Race achieved its purpose.

Like the Dodo bird, Mark seems to be the genius behind the activity in the Blind Center. When I met Mark I was reminded of the old song "Home, home on the range, and the skies are not cloudy all day." For him there is never heard a discouraging word. I came to find out that he had prepared at seminary to become a Southern Baptist preacher. He never explained why he ended up transferring to social work. I am tempted to think that the fundamentalist creed was too alien to his being. He could neither hew Agag in pieces nor preach about such an action, even if commanded by the God of Israel. When students complained that they will have to "graduate" (a nice euphemism that means its quitting time at the Blind Center), Mark reminds that they can always return and join the general classes if they provide their own transportation. As I recall no one seemed to be so presumptuous as to argue with the Dodo bird. And so Mark directs the Caucus Race with equanimity and peace.

I was ushered into an office where a counselor gave me an oral psychological test. I exuded optimism, but rather than being met with a positive response, I could see that the counselor was quite disappointed that I did not need psychological help. The counselor asked me if I were ever suicidal. She added, "Do you ever feel worthless? When you became blind, did you ever feel like crawling into a hole and dying?"

After leaving the Coke machine interview, I wandered around the building, which coincidentally enough did somewhat appear like a race course. In the center of the building is a wide hallway with white squares in the middle and black on either side. Off this hallway on either side are rooms and a few alleys leading elsewhere. I found out that like the Caucus Race, there seemed to be no beginning or ending of this course that the main hallway took. In the words of T. S. Eliot, repeated *ad nauseum*, "In the beginning is my end." So it was that I kept circling the building. Finally in an endeavor to find out how to get out of the place as in Alice's dream, I met a variety of characters moving about in the hallways. There were wheelchairs, there were silent dogs that neither barked nor whined, there were individuals waiving their walking sticks like bewitched enchanters, there were medical walkers, and there were crutches. Through this mix, officious adults moved continually.

Now the Dodo bird prescribed the race with a purpose involved. It is true that no one won or lost exactly, but really everyone won. It is true that students appeared and disappeared with what seemed to be little pattern. Nevertheless, the Dodo bird informed Alice and the menagerie that everybody would win the race. When Alice has problems with deciding what words mean like *glory*, that eminent linguist Humpty Dumpty dictates that the word means whatever he decides it will mean. He does not need to consult any dictionary. So whoever sets up the award system at the Blind Center uses his or her own criteria for judging what words mean. For example, *success* is not judged by any criteria that conventional schools use like examinations and grades. Anyone who stays long enough will graduate with honors, be assured. The honor list has no exceptions. No student is left behind in this race. Every other month graduation exercises take up the entire afternoon with speeches, flowers, and encomiums for the graduates. Actually awards here go by opposites. The more desperate the case of the student, the more he or she is showered with honors. Allen, for example, a young man totally uncoordinated—watch out if he is walking down the hallway as he is swinging his arms and mobility cane in every direction—was highly celebrated at the graduation exercises. Do you know that we found out that he actually learned the letters on the typewriter? In the middle of Kevin's group, he informed the whole assemblage that he had to go to the bathroom. This noble and notable achievement earned him the award of being most improved, and the audience went wild with applause. No Olympic athlete receiving a gold medal ever beamed as Allen did that day. On the other hand, Virginia, who writes good poetry and creates interesting ceramic art, receives little notice.

I realized then that I had failed my interview with the psychologist since I said that I was in a great mental state and that I had no problems. These statements were negatives at the center. How can they rescue the perishing if no one is drowning! Alice finds that the prize she receives is actually a thimble that the Dodo bird had appropriated from her earlier. She receives her own thimble back as a reward. I suppose that the real grade and award comes from one's own self. Your own sense of accomplishment is the prize that you receive. Unfortunately my performance in both Braille and computer class promise no awards since I have given myself a low grade in each. In typing class, however, I performed well and made the teacher happy.

Alice never seemed to ask where all these animals came from. Now while I know how I got to the Blind Center, I have very little idea of how others get there. One man said that his ophthalmologist recommend that he attend. My optometrist didn't recommend for me to attend, nor did my optician, nor my ophthalmologist, nor my retina specialist. My friend Karen and my church friend Troy Potter sent me there.

It is obvious that there are no strict rules about attendance. The other week Salvador arrived with his wife. Kevin urged him with a great deal of earnestness to keep coming back. We have seen neither hide nor hair of Salvador since. Jason, in spite of his body odor, seemed to fit into the program very well. He too disappeareth. My friend Irene found that she had to acquire a fan for her house, and so excused herself for the day. Sadly, Debbie, who attended several weeks, failed to show up on the fourth week. On the fifth week we found out that this middle-aged woman had died. My friend Bob seems to take long absences for "medical reasons." Every week the driver of the bus that transported me to the center calls to see whether or not I am to attend. I expect to follow the rules that I will take the bus unless I call. Apparently the bus driver thinks that I will attend or not depending on what my whims are.

Mark disappears for most of the day. His staff, then, actually assists us in this race. As one moves around in this race, one is helped by the Dodo bird's assistants, whether blind or sighted. None more clearly embody the chief goal of the Blind Center than Kevin, whom I cannot resist calling Kevin the Great. By the way, no one has any last names at the Blind Center. Kevin alone seems really insufficient. How could you call the head of the Round Table as just Arthur, or Norman the Conqueror who invaded England in 1066 as just Norman? Therefore, behind his back I call him Kevin the Great. Perhaps I am thinking of Bunyan's Mr. Great Heart in giving the cognomen "The Great." For some reason I was in Kevin's group for the entire duration of my stay at the Blind Center. I would think that Kevin would shunt me off to another similar group, especially since I know I am prone to talk too much and not let some of the somnolent members respond to Kevin. Kevin's group meets immediately after lunch at 12:45 PM Clarence, the volunteer, arranges the chairs in a circle. I was severely reprimanded when I had rearranged his arrangement. Kevin usually arrives a few minutes late. I said once, "You're late Kevin."

Laughingly, he responded, "Are you going to dock my pay?" Kevin positions himself next to Robert, who has a hearing problem. He then looks at his Braille reader to take attendance. It never fails that some whom he expects to be there are not. Some whom he does not to expect to be there arrive. To each member who answers the roll call, he replies, "I'm glad you're here. I love you all." One time he demonstrated his love by going around the group and hugging everyone—well, the women—and the men got only a token hug. Kevin is likely to begin with, "This is not Kevin's group. It's your group. I'm only the facilitator. I learn from you just as you learn from me."

Kevin then proceeds along to establish tracks. The first is the get-acquainted track. He interviews briefly everyone in the group, but since the group keeps changing, he has to keep interviewing people. He questions the interviewee about when the person went blind, what the nature of the blindness is, and what he or she expects to get out of attendance at the Blind Center. He will then want to know what the ruling passion in the interviewee's life is. Sometimes the interviewees respond that they have no magnificent obsession, whereupon Kevin suggests they get one somewhere. Kevin wants to know also what the person has received from Blind Center.

"Has your attitude been changed towards being blind or have you acquired some skill from any of the classes?"

"Did you find the cooking class helpful?"

"Did Louise in the Assisted Daily Living Class offer you some good tips for coping?"

Scott replied that he had enjoyed eating the cookies made in the cooking class.

The other track is to discover, at great length, the problems or issues facing the group. After each response, Kevin solves the problem with a short statement or a judgment that the issue is a good one. Typical issues are the following: How do I keep other members of my household from moving things around so I can't find them? How can I learn to identify the person to whom I am speaking? What do I say to family members who insist on running my life? How can I find transportation to the grocery store? What do I say to a bus driver who tells me to drop dead? Where can I find help to clean my house? How can I learn to play the piano? Where do I apply if I want to get a guide dog? One woman wanted to know what to do with a nest of eggs she found on her balcony. Irene asked how to open a tin can with the wretched can openers available to her. I could not resist quoting the following: "They are flying now to Mars I hear, but how in the hell do you open a can of beer?" That question did not provide any answers for the dear woman. What do you do when the phone rings and no one answers? How do I get up the courage to ask people to help me out by giving me a ride or giving my mail to me? How can I avoid being struck by a car that whizzes around the corner? How do I respond when people say, "It's over there"? Where is there? I commented that when I asked a bus driver whether his bus went to University Avenue, he said nothing. I happened to notice he was shaking his head. Kevin interlaces his questions with comments like, "You are a very valued member of this group." Kevin asked the group for help in solving these problems, but only after he has solved the problem already.

Now these two approaches of Kevin's sound elemental, but be not deceived: Kevin uses these to inculcate his philosophy of how to cope as a visually handicapped person. He loves to report to the group that Jim and he went cross country skiing for the blind in Colorado. In fact he won one of the races there. No thanks to his first instructor, his second instructor was very helpful. He lards the activities with such admonitions as, "Don't let anyone take away your independence. You can enrich your life by developing new skills." He explains that someone told him he could not write music since he was blind. "I showed him. I've written eight songs with musical scores."

"If you have emotional problems, there is counseling here at the center for you."

"Don't be afraid to ask for help."

"Save your question for the ADL Class."

"Talk to others in the group about how they solve that problem."

"You are not alone; others have faced the same temptations to discouragement that you have faced."

"Think of life as a big orange. There are four areas of life that you need to develop. Divide that orange into four quarters. You need to develop your useful skills first, including holding down a job; two, you need to develop your physical bodies by exercise and diet; three, you need to develop your social skills by being active in community, neighborhood, and church activities; and four, you need to develop your spiritual awareness by worship services, meditation, and inspirational reading." I added that they need to develop their intellectual life, too. Divide that orange up into five pieces.

From the beginning of my days at the Blind Center, I worked not only with Kevin, but with Evelyn, my Braille instructor. While Kevin is Mr. Great Heart, I found that

Evelyn most clearly resembles Alice herself. She gives a lie to every stereotype of the blind as being bold, awkward, useless, and cheerless. That first day when I knocked at her door, a sparkling voice said, "Come in." There sat a beautiful blonde woman whose dress and manners fit the grace of her appearance. I quickly understood why she keeps getting phone calls and people popping in to ask her questions or just chat. In addition to her charm, she exhibits great capability. She is an excellent instructor—clear, orderly, and patient. Every time I said, "I'm a dumbo," she responds with, "No you're not," and goes on with the lesson. I was afraid that when I left the tape recorder with the tape she recorded for me in her office, she would berate me for carelessness. For a whole week I had not studied the lesson she had made for me. Not a bit of it. She went on saying, "Would you like to see my Braille typewriter?" She was delighted when she found out that I wanted to buy a Braille typewriter too. Immediately she located several organizations with which she was familiar and encouraged me to call to find out if they had any used typewriters for sale. New typewriters cost $800. When I expressed my concern over the bus routes, she called the Blind Advocacy Group to enroll me.

I found that Evelyn's quite an amazing woman also outside of the classroom. She is apparently happily married and finds her way all the way from Ramona, a rather distant suburb of San Diego, to the Blind Center with only the help of her mobility cane. I find that she regularly attends the Blind Advocacy Statewide Convention and for some years was a Braille editor. Thankfully, she reflects the Center's philosophy and tells me not to worry about performing poorly. Nevertheless, I did not want to show her how weak my performance was. Can you imagine the frustration of trying to figure out whether the configuration of dots is an *r* or *w*? One strategy I use to prevent her from finding out how poorly I am reading Braille is to distract her from observing my progress by bringing up some new subject of conversation. She is rather easily led astray because she has a wide interest in many subjects. I got her talking about the bus route changes, preparedness for a terrorist attack, the volunteer next door whom I met at the university, and traveling in Europe.

Goodness knows she tries all kinds of devices to enable me to learn. For a while she switched me to jumbo Braille. It is an unfortunate term since I keep thinking of jumbo and dumbo together. What has proved helpful, and I tell her so, is to read my textbook while I record her voice. Then I can follow with my finger the words she is reading. One time she said, "I'll tell you what. I'll lend you a Braille typewriter, but don't tell anyone else that I'm doing it."

No teacher has helped me so much as Lisa, the mobility instructor. When I first arrived at her cubicle, I waited until she appeared with sandwich in hand. The first class of our session she looked at my wooden walking stick as if it had been a dead rat. "I like my stick," I said. "I swing it when I cross the road and use it to feel the way in front of me. I'm afraid that if I got a mobility cane I might be mugged." While chewing on the sandwich, Lisa responded with disdain, "Here are three mobility canes. You *will* pick one and buy it. You *will* use the mobility cane and throw away that wooden stick." I no more had the courage to resist Lisa's orders than I had to disobey the hookah-smoking caterpillar. It was absolutely settled: I would start using a mobility cane.

The most difficult class to which I was assigned was the computer class. Mark was quite pleased to announce that he had secured me a place in the class. To enter the class I had to leave the Caucus Room Building and enter an adjacent building by a yellow brick sidewalk. I thought perhaps I was going to enter the Land of Oz because certainly the world of computers is as strange as Dorothy's world. But I found that the computer class had not departed from the world of Alice's Wonderland, only the Caucus Race part of it.

What I found was that the computer class most nearly resembled the croquet game in the Queen of Hearts' garden. Cathy and Carl ruled this garden. Cathy would sit in the office and occasionally yell out instructions to Carl, sometimes contradicting his instructions. When I got so mixed up that I stopped typing on the computer hooked up to the JAWS program, she entered to command, "Off with his head!" Actually she simply said, "How did you get yourself in this mess?" Now Carl turned out to be a very nice man and a patient man, but operated under two constraints. The first was the interference occasioned by Cathy's intrusions into the process, and second was the problem with the instructional tapes which were not coordinated with the computer. Carl would tell me one set of instructions, but these instructions disappeared as much as Alice's hedgehog croquet balls crept away. While Carl told me to turn on the JAWS program simply by pressing the windows key and J, the tapes said to press the control key and J. While Carl said to press the windows key and M to find my document, the tape said to press the lower arrow until I located my file. I felt as baffled as when Alice's croquet mallet turned out to be a flamingo that refused to cooperate with her efforts. The poor man was stuck with inadequate and outdated equipment.

On the Caucus Race course, in addition to the Dodo and his accomplices, there were the fellow racers as varied as the mouse, the duck, the eaglet, and the lorry. When I first entered the Blind Center, everybody looked generally the same: white-haired and elderly. While they lacked the immediate appeal that young people possess, I found that they were perhaps more interesting than young people when you got to know them. I could talk of Irene, the ninety-one year old lady that rode with me on the bus to the Center. We liked to tease her by asking her what she had in her lunch sack for us. Since she took the same cooking class that we took, we asked for brownies. Every week her answer was the same. She had packed a half of cheese sandwich. The news caused us to moan. When I would say, "What classes do you have today, Irene?" She would say, "I don't know." Beside her family her poodle seems to occupy most of her concern: she wonders if it would be too hot waiting for her on the porch. Her only wish that I could detect was that someone would take her dancing.

Bob should really take her up on that since he is the same age. He lives in an efficiency apartment in Hillcrest. Why he has no female escort I don't know since he is always talking about pretty women. His clever and constant sarcasm hides probably an idealist. He would offer to take over the job of driving the van or ask the driver to take us to Blacks nudist beach instead of the Center.

The most remarkable student that I've met was Janet. The first day of class I met Janet in Kevin's group. Elizabeth Bowen describes the poet Edith Sitwell in her eccentricity as "a high altar on the move." I can best describe Janet as a one-person show on the move. She reminds me of a street performer that plays the harmonica, a banjo, and a drum at the same time and sports a monkey on an organ grinder. Janet sat in a wheelchair with a mobility cane and a harnessed Labrador named Magic by her side. A sign on the dog tells the viewer that it is not a seeing-eye dog, but a guide dog. Therefore, I enjoy petting Magic. What startled me was that Janet spoke to the group with a deep man's voice. I wasn't sure at first where the voice came from. I finally realized that she could not speak and was typing the message into a mechanical device. Now why the makers of such devices can't have other voice alternatives than a deep man's voice I don't know. Perhaps they are not aware that women can lose their voices as well as men.

One day Janet sat against the wall crying. Her daughter had told her that since she was a blind old woman no one would bother to listen to her. Quickly, Troy Potter, the man who had invited me to the center in the first place, rushed over to comfort her. I might add that the same Troy Potter took the trouble to visit the hundred-year-old student at his home one week before he died. For nine months I did not see Janet since I was teaching overseas. When I returned to Kevin's group, there was Janet in wheelchair with her mobility cane and her dog Magic. A beautiful mellifluous woman's voice spoke up. I couldn't believe that Janet was speaking with her own voice instead of that mechanical masculine voice.

Kevin told the story of her transformation. She had accompanied Kevin and several other blind students to a rally in Downtown San Diego for the rights of the handicapped. In the middle of one of the speeches, Janet became so enthusiastic she shouted out, "Yes!" It was the first word she had uttered in years, and she never stopped talking in her beautiful voice since. I was reminded of the 19th century Thomas Carlyle's chapter on "The Everlasting Yea." Like Janet, Carlyle had undergone deep distress over what he saw as the meaninglessness of a mechanical world without God or a purpose—a world of the everlasting no. Struggling with his despair on a wild Scottish farm, Carlyle mustered his spirit to utter the everlasting yea.

When Janet graduated from the Center for the Blind, she exemplified her yes with a desire to return to the Center as a volunteer to teach an alternative Braille system that she was excited about. That yes by Janet articulated best all the talk at the San Diego Center for the Blind. All the instructors were saying yes. And as I sat around the long tables where we had our opening exercises and our lunch, I heard the students saying, "Yes, yes, and yes."

Although it is easy to poke fun at the Blind Center's resemblance to a Caucus Race, like Alice's Caucus Race, the Blind Center does accomplish the goal that the Dodo bird promised. The Caucus Race did manage to dry everyone off from the wetness of the pool of tears. Mark, with his laid-back strategy, actually achieves something quite marvelous. I call it the fellowship of the journey. On a broader scale, in life, perhaps the greatest benefit of living is this fellowship of the journey. After all, is the meaning of life to be judged only by what diplomas hang on our walls and what positions of authority we have achieved? Is not the fellowship with other human beings, with animals, and with nature a chief purpose in life? Lewis Auchincloss in the novel *The Rector of Justin* portrays a famous headmaster looking back at his career as educator and forgetting all of the honorary degrees and fame in assessing his career states, "I think I have helped a few students." And frankly, what is more rewarding than working and playing with family and co-workers and acquaintances in the fellowship of the journey? The journey itself has little value. So it's not surprising that the real value of the Center for the Blind Caucus Race is the fellowship of the journey.

One student recorded that after she lost her vision, she sat pitying herself, isolated in her room. After coming to the Blind Center, she discovered that she was not alone; that a lot of people have vision problems; that they laugh and joke and learn to manage to cope with the cards that have been dealt them. If there is one overriding atmosphere at the Blind Center it is of happiness and fun. I think that my own reluctance in obtaining a mobility cane arose at least partially from a feeling that I would appear as some speckled bird. After attending the Blind Center, I feel like a representative of a wonderful group of people who are resourceful and positive in living. I know that at the Blind Center we are taught skills, but frankly most of us are too old to worry about a career. Our main career at this point is living, and living with some degree of independence, optimism, and even joy.

Chapter Three:

Eyeless in Chicago

To illustrate what one encounters in daily life if one is visually handicapped, I will relate my adventures in another wonderland, aka: Chicago's Union Terminal. Like most modern buildings, it is very difficult to tell the head from the tail. Is it not true, for example, that many stores endeavor to keep shoppers in as long as possible and to make an exit from the store an act of divination? The taxi from the hotel let me off at an entrance, one of a number, I guessed. I had broken up my journey from Syracuse, New York to San Diego, California by a one-day's stay at the Palmer House Hotel. As I approached the doors, I wondered whether they would open automatically or which ones would operate open-by-hand. Once inside, I saw stairs ascending and stairs descending.

Since I was hungry, I decided to look for a lunch counter. I tried the steps going up and proceeded to run into a glass wall. Fortunately my head is hard and my body firm, and I quickly recovered my composure. I guessed where the counter was and saw a shape behind the counter that I took to be a clerk. "What's on the menu?" I asked.

"Just look above the counter," a voice responded.

"You'll have to tell me," I said. "I can't see well enough to read." I ordered a sandwich and coffee. Behind me were machines where I was to fill my own coffee. I guessed at which one was the decaffeinated machine and fumbled around trying to discover how to operate it. Should I find a metal lever under the tab and push it, or should I place the cup under the tab and press the tab? By the way, which tab was which? Might I get ice water, 7-Up, hot chocolate, hot water, plain water, regular coffee, or decaffeinated coffee? I got something hot and brown and settled for its approximation to what I wanted. After every burst from the nozzle, I checked to see how full it was. Spoons, forks, napkins, cream, sugar, and condiments lay in a great blur also on the counter. The waitress took my twenty-dollar bill and then handed me some bills in change, a receipt, and some coins all in one swift gesture, leaving me to sort out the mess. I carried my change, sandwich, packets of condiments, coffee, and plastic silverware over to a table. The sandwich was encased in a plastic container, which had been taped together. I fumbled to see which side opened. It proved to be the wrong side. I attacked the other side, but the Scotch tape held firmly. Grabbing a plastic fork, I inserted it under the tape, but the prong of the fork broke off before it could loosen the tape. The knife finished the operation, and I opened the container. I have learned to be wary of toothpicks stuck into the sandwich to hold them together. Beside the sandwich were, I discovered, a pickle, an olive, and a small container of salsa. My finger came away bedecked with the red stuff. After drinking and eating my fill, I looked around for the can in which to place my trash. Observing none, I left the mess on the counter. I did not run into the glass door again, but proceeded through another set of glass doors to what I thought would be the main terminal which I had seen before. It was an elegant waiting room with huge classical pillars, but with very few people. They were all crammed below in cubicles. As soon as I passed through the doors, a burly guard wanted to know what I was up to. Perhaps my luggage contained a bomb or machine gun. "I am looking for the waiting room," I responded.

"This is not the waiting room. This is an office building," he said. How had Union Station morphed into an office building, I wondered. But I retreated, and in the guard's mind, perhaps saved the structure from collapse.

Once outside the office building, I headed down two flights of stairs to a subterranean midden that rivals Kings Cross Station in London, where I warn any visually handicapped person to avoid like the plague. I got caught in the entrails of this behemoth once and managed to find my way out to the street, whereupon I was approached by a stranger who said, "I am lost. Can you give me directions for the main entrance to this station?"

I responded, "You couldn't possibly have found a worse person to ask directions than the one you have just asked since I am half blind and lost myself." Although I realized that there were lots of little signs around, I could read none, and there was no official person standing there. Commuters were rushing around me and did not welcome any interruption. There were waiting rooms everywhere, all looking identical. The railroad tracks appeared through glass doors with a constant cacophony of voices announced trains arriving on Track 16 and 18 and departing on 24. I thought of the maze at the Isle of Crete or of Kafka's castle. Two guards were lounging on some go-carts, engaged in hearty camaraderie.

"Where is the main Amtrak waiting-room?" I asked. Finally I caught the attention of one of the men. He waved his arm, I thought, toward the right. Lo and behold! There appeared, apparently, an information desk. After waiting for the disposal of three customers, the attendant told me to proceed forward, take a right, and then take the first left.

I discovered a ticket counter—perhaps the Amtrak ticket counter.

"Where is the main waiting room?" I asked.

"Across the way," she replied.

"Could I have a little more definite direction? I don't see well," I said.

"Do you see that silver pillar?" she said.

"Not really," I said truthfully.

"Do you see those white carts?" she asked.

"Honestly, I don't," I replied.

"Wait here. I'll call a red cap," she said. Ten minutes later, a red cap appeared and offered to take me to the waiting room.

"Grab hold of my arm," he instructed.

"No. I can follow you," I said. In truth, the waiting room was only a stone's throw away. Leading me to the first row of chairs, he approached a middle-aged lady, instructing her to help me since I was blind. No mother ever received an adopted child with more solicitation than did this poor soul. Every twenty minutes she asked me how I was doing. "Fine," I said. She informed me that she grew up in Jamaica. When I showed her my book of memoirs, she replied that she would like to write her own life. Having wearied of listening to tapes, I pulled out a piece of paper and pen, placing the paper on the same book of memoirs, and started writing about the train station. Now, when I write away from my typewriter, I know that the writing will be unreadable, since I write over what I have written very often. Her sharp eye noticed this problem. So what seemed a peculiarly obvious gambit, she proceeded to lean over me to grab my hand and move it down to the next line. As soon as my pen would move, she was on top of me, warning me that I was writing over what I had already written. Now this great guide to international travel informed me that she had missed the train the day before. Yet she was to make sure that I found my train. I began to wonder whether she was really waiting for a train or hosting some kind of party since people started emerging from the crowd to greet her as a long-lost friend or neighbor. How could she know so many people in this terminal? I wondered. Now to her credit, she did take my money to buy me a coke and would not buy one with my money for herself. Soon when she was busy greeting all these people, I escaped to the restroom. I began to feel that I was in the way of all her guests and so seated myself two rows from her. Soon she spotted me, however, and asked me whether I was doing okay. Where I really needed help was to find the right line for the train I was to take. The station was packed with people, and when the announcer called for those who were over sixty-two and handicapped, I had no idea where the line was. I couldn't see the number of the gate at all and finally had to jump over a chair to locate the gate. Just when I needed her, of course, she had vanished. Whether she had caught her train or whether she was greeting her many friends, I knew not.

An announcement came over the loud speaker, "The Southwest Chief will be late because of engine trouble." What does late mean, I wondered? Five minutes, fifteen minutes, or five hours? Distinct from the hot, stuffy waiting room where I had been ensconced for several hours, the waiting area for the handicapped was cold and breezy. I contemplated what I should do, whether I should use the restroom during this protracted session. I shuddered at the thought of going past the security guards and plowing my way through the mass of people that were waiting inside the terminal. I wondered if I could find my way back out to the waiting area. Fortunately after an hour, people started leaving the waiting area for the train, even though no announcement ever informed us that the train was then ready. I walked down the long ramp, avoiding carts and piles of luggage and hoping not to step on a black garment bag being pulled before me. My troubles all disappeared as I made my way to the dining car and was seated to be served a delicious turkey dinner. It was 8:00 PM before this blessed event took place, but this meal was worth waiting for. I breathed a sigh of relief to be on the train, where there was only one hallway. If I walked forward, I would without fail walk into the lounge car and then the dining car. In the dining car, the hostess would seat me at a table, and a waiter or waitress would bring food and drinks to me. If I counted the cars between the lounge and my sitting car, I would be sure to find my seat. From Chicago to Los Angeles, my life would be simple, organized, and secure. Goodbye, I thought, to that mass of wriggling humanity in this center of the nation. I remembered the slogan from years ago, "A hog can cross the country without changing trains, but you can't." Chicago terminal awaits all transcontinental passengers, although it keeps its old glories as a monument and subjects its present customers to an ordeal of loud television, cell phones, constant reminders to check for suspicious behavior, and illegible signs for the visually handicapped.

CHAPTER FOUR:

The Swallower of Serpents

When Moses received the order from the Almighty to confront Pharaoh, he complained of his inadequacy. The writer of Exodus records God asking, "What is that in thy hand?" Moses must have replied that it is a walking stick of some sort. God said, "Throw it down." To his astonishment, Moses saw the stick morph into a serpent. When he picked the nasty thing up by its tail, it again became a stick. With this trick, Moses confronted the king. Not to be outdone, the king's magicians threw their sticks on the ground, which also became serpents. Moses had the last laugh because his snake swallowed up the serpents of the magicians.

In similar fashion my mobility cane has swallowed up all my entire collection of walking sticks. Now when I became blind, I didn't hear any supernatural voice ordering me to buy a mobility cane, although my brother Stephen, who from my early childhood tried to play the role of God, commanded me to get one. I am ashamed to say that for about ten years I wandered around the wilderness with many walking sticks like the magicians' serpents of inferior quality to the mobility cane. Although I love walking sticks, they possess none of the magical quality that the mobility cane possesses.

When I was using plain walking sticks, upon asking bus drivers the number of the route, they seemed to sometimes resent telling me. "Look," said one burly son of Malach. When I explained that I was legally blind, he shook his fist at me. I asked another driver, who stood beside the open door of his bus, whether the vehicle was the number 10 bus. He remained totally silent. You see, the walking sticks that I used failed to tell the world that I was handicapped. Perhaps they thought that I was lame or addicted to the whimsy of flourishing a walking stick.

I'm not sure why I resisted switching to the white mobility cane. I am attached to my collection of walking sticks. My favorite was created and given to me by one of my former students, Byron Hoot, who is also a member of the Tamarack Writers Group. One July day, without ceremony, he took away the feeble stick I had bought at the Old Forge Hardware, and stuck in my hand the clean white rod he had fashioned the year before, taken from the spot where we sit by the lake and read our creations. The stick is capped by a leather handle and strap. I asked all the writers there to sign their names, and although their names have faded, in my mind they are there still. My next favorite stick is an ivory headed one. The ivory cap had three sides, celebrating the great British naval hero, Lord Nelson. On one side is the ship, the *H.M.S. Victory*, a ship that led the English to success in the Battle of Trafalgar. On one of the other sides is a portrait of Lord Nelson himself. On the third side appears his coat of arms. While I was in the JFK airport headed for Europe, a man tried to purchase my walking stick that twisted like a snake or a screw. It was reminiscent of the serpentine stick in Hawthorne's "Young Goodman Brown." Stubbornly I refused to sell the stick.

My resistance to using the magic mobility cane ended at the San Diego Center for the Blind. I was sent to Lisa for mobility training. As I have mentioned before, she disapproved of my walking stick and, opening a closet that resembled a storage space for skeletons, said. "Take your pick." There were some real monstrosities there. Some with curved handles and one with three prongs at the bottom, designed for people who may topple over at any moment. I would have nothing to do with canes with curved tops or with triple prongs. I identify such things with aged crones slipping into the grave, creeping along life's pathway emitting auras of grey depression around them. Rather, I picked the fairest of the lot— one that resembles a ski pole or a mountain climbing stick. "I'll buy that stick," I said. While pulling it out of the closet, Lisa sternly corrected my language, "It is not a walking stick. It is a *mobility cane.*"

I don't like calling it a cane in the first place. In the second case, the term *mobility cane* was dreamed up by some politically correct social worker. Another politically correct term that I dislike is *visually handicapped* or *visually challenged.* Hey folks, I'm legally blind; that is half blind. You don't hurt my feelings by saying that I'm legally blind. Such politically correct terminology is used for death. *Passed away* is bad enough, but *passed* is beyond the pail. I associate the term either with passing gas or passing a course. Occasionally someone will ask me, "Do you mind talking about your eye problem?"

"I don't mind a bit," I respond. "I'm not ashamed of the fact that I am legally blind and appreciate your interest in me." I wish someone would interview me on NPR or on a late night talk show.

Lisa set about showing me the magic qualities of the mobility cane. As I waited for her to appear on the second day, I examined this new artifact. I found out that it must be white. At the bottom of the white cane is a foot of colored red. At the base of the cane is a round rolling white ball. At the top of the cane is a black rubbery handle, which I later found is the same used in golf clubs. At the top is a cord that binds the cane together when it is folded into five sections. Two elastic cords keep the cane together when it is folded. As I looked at the folded cane, I realized that it would make a good club to beat off any muggers. When Lisa appeared she asked, "Why did you wait ten years before buying a mobility cane?" I was on trial to explain my foolishness.

"Let's see," I said. "I associate blindness with old age, and I wish to appear to be thirty three even though I am over twice that age. Next," I averred, "I was fearful that I would invite muggers, who would think that I could not identify them because of my blindness." My third excuse was simply that I was a victim of inertia. How many things do we have on our list of what we ought to do, but won't do until we are impelled to do so!

I minored in history during my undergraduate days. I'm not sure why I feel like a stranger when I don't know the history of the place where I happen to be. Can you really be an American without knowing something of American history? What richness the past brings to the present. I therefore think that it's important to know a little history about the white mobility cane. Of course, shepherd staffs have been used since ancient days. In addition to herding sheep, they developed to being used by travelers even if no sheep were around. Mountain climbers found that these staffs aided in ascending steep places. I'm sure that the blind found these staffs helpful in moving around, keeping one from falling down, or running into an object. Like so many artifacts of civilization, it appears that the white cane itself did not become a symbol for the blind until the 20th century. What in the world were people doing the previous 6,000 years of civilization? Awake ye sleepers of the night!

A little history reveals that the mobility cane was not the creation of some politically correct social worker. The first record that we have of the white cane being used to identify a blind person was that of a certain artist in Bristol named James Biggs. After this artist became blind through an accident, he painted his walking cane white in order to maneuver the increasing traffic that he faced in his walks, knowing that no regular walking stick is white. Perhaps we find here in this fact a clue. We can blame the evolution of the mobility cane on Henry Ford and his infernal invention, a threat to all the blind. It's one thing to step out of the way when you hear the clomp of horse hooves and wheels; it's something else when one of Henry Ford's behemoths comes roaring at you at sixty miles an hour as some do even on city streets. Why, when Prince Albert found that the horseless carriage he was riding on exceeded twenty miles an hour, he ordered the train to slow down, fearing that such rapid speed could not be conducive to good health. I wish to insert in this narrative a fact that the sound of vehicles helps me to avoid them. Recently an owner of a hybrid car bragged that his vehicle could appear on the scene without any noise. That's just what we blind people need—a noiseless car mowing us down, knocking us all over like tenpins. If commercial trucks trigger a beeper when they move in reverse, certainly we will need some kind of warning from these hybrid cars.

It wasn't until the thirties that groups decided to promote the use of the white cane for blind pedestrians. In 1931, Guilly d'Herbemont began a movement for recognizing the white cane as a symbol for the blind. On hearing of Guilly d'Herbemont's movement, the British Rotary Club promoted a similar idea throughout the British Empire. The BBC also promoted the use of the white mobility cane.

After this, the Lions Club has taken a special interest in the blind.

In the United States, it took until 1937 before the mobility cane began to be legalized as protection for the blind. At this time an ordinance was passed in the state of Michigan giving the bearers of mobility canes precedence in their movement over other moving objects. Momentum for recognition of the mobility cane was increased by the return of veterans who had become blind during World War II. Finally in 1960 congress made the mobility cane an official symbol for the blind throughout the whole country and established October 15th as Mobility Cane Day. Unfortunately Congress did not dictate that this day of recognition should be celebrated by fireworks or parades. To tell the truth, I didn't discover the fact until I "Googled" it in my computer.

Lisa explained that the mobility cane is partly magic in itself and partly magic in how it is used. She didn't need to tell me that the cane shouldn't be thrust in front of one awkwardly, as if one is in a duel. At the Blind Center, we have another living example of how not to use the mobility cane. Robert walked down the hallway flailing both arms and mobility cane, as if doing the breast stroke, or better yet flailing as if he were trying to keep from drowning. Down the aisles of the Blind Center, Lisa instructed me to roll the mobility cane back and forth, at the width of ones body. The cane should hit the right side of the aisle, thus letting you know when there are doorways. How nicely the cane rolled along the aisles of the San Diego Center for the Blind. Then Lisa took me outdoors. Again I was to roll the cane on the sidewalk. Instead of hitting the end of the wall, one should hit the end of the sidewalk as it met the grass. Arriving at an intersection, Lisa told me to perch at the edge of the curb my feet half on and half off the curb. If I were to fall, she informed me that she would catch me in her capacious arms. Perhaps I should have tried her out to see if she really would catch me.

Now Lisa was fully sighted, and her instruction was perfectly correct—that is in an ideal world. But friends, we do not live in an ideal world, I'm sorry to tell you. It's one thing to roll the cane on the smooth halls of the Blind Center. It's another thing to roll the thing on the cracked and uneven sidewalks of the city away from the Blind Center. Try rolling the cane on a gravel path. Now Lisa's instructions are perfectly good for a perfectly blind person. However, I am not going to go waving my cane in front of me when I can see what is in front of me perfectly well if the light is proper. One observer noted, "You walk as if you know where you're going." The more confidently I walk, the more I will intimidate highwaymen and robbers. Sometimes if the light is right, I use my mobility cane as a walking stick. Sometimes I hold it in the middle, since I am fairly confident of the path in front of me. At other times, I fold the cane up completely. When one walks on city streets, the light often changes to shadow, and there I need the extended mobility cane. At night I always use the cane extended. Now wouldn't it be my luck to find that Lisa caught me using the mobility cane in an unauthorized manner. How was I to know that she would be in North Park training a student three miles from the Blind Center? Well as a child we sang a chorus, "Be careful little feet where you go." The reason for being careful is that the Almighty is always watching. I was confident that Lisa was not possessed with the attribute of omnipresence—too confident as it turns out. What Lisa did not talk to me about was not the practicality of the mobility cane, but the artistry of its use. You can't use a saw effectively until you love the saw. The mobility cane is not used effectively until you see it as an object of beauty and grace.

Years before while working for my college roommate's father in Cleveland, Ohio, he informed me that I was fighting the saw that I was attempting to use. He commented, "You mean to tell me that you have finished three years of college and still don't know how to use a saw?" I should have answered, "I am afraid that I failed Sawing 101 in my sophomore year." Certainly one should not fight the mobility cane. Not only should the mobility cane be aesthetically pleasing, but the handling of it should be graceful and artistic. I can recall one poor blind young man who jabbed the mobility cane forward in a helter-skelter kind of fashion, resembling a drowning man attempting to swim.

When I was in the army, we learned to handle our M1 rifle with respect and dignity. An instructor informed us that in battle, your rifle is your best friend. He recounted a previous session in which to his statement that "the rifle is your best friend in battle," a trainee objected asserting, "The rifle is not your best friend in battle; Jesus Christ is." I'm sure that the instructor was willing to concede that the M1 rifle is your second best friend in battle, behind Jesus Christ.

The rifle became part of our military presence. There were rules for its handling when one was on parade or in formation. We were instructed to service our rifle by oiling it down before we retired for the night. How disillusioned I was when the squad leader who gave us this instruction, and who was my tent mate, entered the tent on a rainy night and threw the wet rifle, oilless, beside his sleeping bag. We were told that when we were "at ease," our left hand was placed at the small of our back. The butt of the rifle rested by our right foot, and our right hand was extended so that the rifle jutted forward at an angle. When the officer called attention, our left hand moved to our side, and the left foot moved to the right foot. The right hand brought the rifle along the right side of one's body. With the command "present arms," the right hand lifted the rifle to the center of the body while the left hand grasped the rifle beneath the right hand. With the command "order arms," the left hand fell to the side of the body, and the right hand brought the rifle back to the right hand side. With the command "right shoulder arms," the right hand brought the rifle in front of the body at an angle while the left arm grasped the rifle beneath the right hand. The left hand then moved to the butt of the rifle while the right hand brought the rifle to ones shoulder. At the final movement, the left hand returned to the side of the left leg. Of course, the rifle always was required to be immaculately clean. The wood was polished, and the metal was oiled. Elite units showed off their skill by tossing their rifles to each other, or, if there were four soldiers performing, to one another. They twirled the rifles like batons and threw them into the air to be caught. How much more agile is the mobility cane! I can twirl mine with both the left hand and the right hand. Often I fold up the mobility cane while I'm sitting on a bus. When I am about to stand up, I unleash the strap, and with a quick movement hold the cane up in the air while it unfolds itself. The trick is to let the mobility cane unfold with a minimum of noise and with one movement of the arm. If one performs this action quickly and gracefully, one need not startle other passengers by its unfolding. In all my fancy maneuvering of the mobility cane, I have to restrain myself. It makes an excellent pointer, except for the fact that people don't like to be jabbed by a pointer. And the mobility cane has a long reach. The other morning, I was whirling the mobility cane and hit my colleague in the head with my cane. Art has its limits.

If you love your mobility cane, or anything else, it will not remain nameless to you. Martin Buber points out that

I-thou is much more significant than I-it. I trust, dear reader, that you do not drive a car that is nameless. Cars operate better when they are named. We in America tend to live in houses that are unnamed. How do you think the house feels when you call it "357 Oak Street?" When I was driving from Bristol to Exeter, I wished to see the place where Coleridge went to visit the Wordsworths after he had met Wordsworth at a lecture in Bristol. Stopping at a service station along the way, I inquired to the attendant, "Could you tell me how to get to Racedown?"

Looking puzzled he said, "Sir, I have operated this station for twenty years and have never heard of the town Racedown." At the moment, an old twenties vintage Bentley drove into the station, and a tall dignified man unbent himself. The attendant said, "Ask that man where Racedown is. If he doesn't know, no one knows."

I approached the dignified elder. "Sir, could you tell me where the town Racedown is?"

Looking a bit startled, he said, "Racedown? That's not a town; that's a house," and proceeded to give me the most particular directions through one-laned roads and curves to the place in question. I named my house in Ohio "Twin Firs" since it had two huge trees in front of it. Anyway, I decided to name my mobility cane "Tam" after that venerable traveler described by Robert Burns, namely Tam O' Shanter.

Moses was able to use his staff not only to impress Pharaoh, but to do wonderful things like parting the Red Sea. The Children of Israel, after escaping from Egypt supposedly to have a religious celebration, heard that the armies of Pharaoh were advancing on them, and before them was the Red Sea. In this most difficult situation, Moses stretched out his staff so that the Israelites could walk through to the other side. Pharaoh's chariots, of course, pursued them. But, when they were in the middle of the sea bed, Moses raised his staff again and the waters covered them. Now I have been unable to part the sea with my mobility cane, but I have parted traffic, stopping huge trucks and busses while I walked across roads with perfect safety. I must concede that the mobility cane, as good as its magic is, lacks the authority that Moses' cane possessed. Sometimes I part traffic, but I must not presume that I will always do so.

To tell the truth, this mobility cane is not always as effective as it should be. Recently a truck zoomed around University Avenue onto Kansas Street. It so happens that I was walking across Kansas Street. Fortunately I saw the oncoming truck and stopped. How did the driver know that I can see quite a bit and am not totally blind? If I had not stopped, he would either have slammed on his brakes or toppled me over.

My mobility cane has not been quite so effective on sidewalks. Sometimes pedestrians avoid me, but sometimes I have to jump out of their way. Perhaps I should just stick the cane under their feet and trip them up to teach them a lesson. My poor friend Bob had his mobility cane run over by a wheelchair. Apparently wheelchairs take precedence over mobility canes. Generally the mobility cane works its magic, making bus drivers tell me where to sit, forcing people to give up their seats for me (which actually I do not really wish), and letting the whole world know that I am visually handicapped. Therefore, the whole society around me understands my movements and usually offers me their assistance.

Just yesterday I was walking on the platform at the trolley station in Old Town, and a young man came rushing towards me asking if I was okay. I assured him that I was, but thanked him for his concern. Now I have been constantly puzzled by the scarceness of the mobility cane. On the route seven bus that passes the Blind Center on Upas Street, I often see the white cane, but often I go days without seeing another one. Only one other person at church had a mobility cane, but he has moved away. As many times as I have gone to the Old Globe Theatre at Balboa Park, I have yet to see anyone else with a white cane. Do the blind not attend the theatre? I have traveled extensively in Western Europe. In Italy I have not observed a single walking cane. In London and Paris I have seen a few. I challenge you: have you ever seen a mobility cane in an art gallery? Unless you see me behind a mobility cane, you have probably not seen a mobility cane. On a student trip to Vienna, I approached an entrance to an art gallery. A student that accompanied me informed the door keeper that I was blind. Apparently he had never been told what to do if a blind person tried to enter the museum. In his befuddlement, he waved me through without charging a Euro. One can't blame the young boy in the Underground in London for looking at my walking cane intently. The poor boy was scolded by his father who said, "Don't stare." Dear dad, how in the world would I know if the kid was staring at the mobility cane, and furthermore I wouldn't care. And furthermore, dad should have used the occasion to explain the significance of the mobility cane.

On a vaparetto from Lido to the main islands of Venice, a little boy sitting on his mother's lap could not keep himself from grabbing the cane. When his mother tried to stop him, I smiled and said it was okay. I even let him handle the strap on top. In spite of the language barrier, I found that he was three years old, and his name was Salvador. When mother and child got up to leave, she had him give me a little peck on the cheek.

Not only small children fail to understand the significance of the mobility cane, a certain bewhiskered lush, holding up the Rome train station on seeing me pass with my mobility cane, wanted to know if I was going skiing. A similar creature in San Diego wanted to know if I were going mountain climbing. I responded to both, "I am neither going skiing nor mountain climbing, but I am faring forth in this dark world with a magical stick which has more power and wonder in it than the best ski pole in the world, or those special mountain sticks used to climb Mt. Everest."

Chapter Five:

The Big Bang and I

Part 1: Physical Aspects of Color

Like lobsters being boiled, the awareness of the increasing heat of their environment probably dawns on them slowly. Eventually they begin complaining loudly, but at first they are probably enjoying the nice warmth of the water as one might enjoy sitting by a fire on a winter's evening. The slow decline of my eyes is often not even noticeable. Then suddenly I am aware that I see differently than I had previously.

As I have stated elsewhere, the discovery of my disability occurred at first slowly, and then dramatically. At first I was diagnosed by my ophthalmologist as having macular degeneration. Then a specialist changed that diagnosis to Retinitis Pigmentosa. That retina specialist mysteriously disappeared (perhaps he vanished from sight), and the next diagnosis I received was that of Stargardt's disease. The final diagnosis, like the first, was that of age-related macular degeneration, and I feel sure that this is the correct diagnosis. In a way, it was disappointing to receive this diagnosis since it is very common to mankind, especially to older people. Everybody has age-related macular degeneration. My understanding is that in the macula, or center part of the eye, the tissue thins and degenerates, clogging the light receptors (cones and rods) with material from the thinning tissue.

The result of this deterioration is that it is especially hard to read or to see people's faces. I have to ask people who they are. I say "Who's that?" quite loudly and without any hesitation. Of course sometimes I can tell who's speaking to me by the tone of his/her voice or some distinguishing physical characteristic. But when girls wear men's shirts and pants, and when boys wear long hair and pony tails, I sometimes get the genders wrong. Even before my eyes fell into disrepair, I asked a young woman in the front row of my class who she was. I had not remembered a dark haired girl in the front row before. It turned out that she was the cute blonde girl who had dyed her hair the previous night. One of my Japanese students dyed her hair green, much to the distress of her parents back in Japan. I was complaining about the inability of identifying attendants at the desk of the fitness center since several young ladies rotated at the post. My instructor at the Blind Center told me to ask them who they are. I followed his suggestion, and they didn't seem to mind. Now actually, my inability to identify people has its bright side. If an old student from the dark ages comes up to me expecting to know his or her name, I say, holding my mobility cane, "Oh, I can't see who you are. Who are you?" When they give me their names, I act as if, of course, that I remember them. Well, it's an ill wind that does not bring some good.

Recently my assistant Marilyn "Googled" a macular degeneration article. They showed on the screen beneath a regular picture one that illustrated what a person with macular degeneration sees. She gasped and exclaimed, "I can't see their faces."

"Just so. Now you know," I replied.

I hated giving up driving. Every visually impaired person I know has had the same reaction. The driving of an automobile is almost a right guaranteed in the constitution as an inalienable right. What red-blooded American can surrender his or her right to drive a car? I imagined that trying to ride a city bus was an adventure in madness. I didn't know where the bus stops were! I imagined that the busses ran on an erratic time schedule. I wondered whether I would be imprisoned in my own home because I could not get around. I could see myself standing forlornly on the street, waiting for a bus that never came. How could I shop, recreate, and work with no car? Of course I panicked at the thought that I could not read, especially because I am a literature and language teacher. I worried about crossing streets, traveling on airplanes, and finding literary places in Great Britain all without the aid of good eyes. In reality, I tend to brag about how I have adjusted to my vision loss on all of these subjects. However, there are countless frustrations and limitations that my impairment has on my physical maneuverability.

Like the lobsters being boiled, I began to realize that I wasn't seeing colors as I used to. It came as a jolt when I recognized that the trees and the grass were now black, or at least charcoal. I suppose that in poor light trees become black (especially at night); I simply did not notice that even in bright light they had become black. I decided that I must take inventory of my vision to find out just what I could see and what I could not. As of recent days people constantly wonder what kind of visual landscape I experience. It is not easy to describe exactly what I do see. I don't even try to look at distance objects and since I am near sighted, I stopped wearing my glasses altogether! What is the point of trying to see objects accurately at a distance? Hurray, I'm free of glasses! At first I experienced mild eye aches when I did not wear my glasses. Gradually my eyes adjusted. And I am sure I must look much handsomer. Certainly I no longer have to hunt for them. Several times I have been looking for my glasses when they were actually on my face.

My usual explanation for what I can see and what I can not see is that there seems to be a fog over everything—a fog that keeps me from seeing anything distinctly. I understand a verse in the Bible through this experience. The Gospel writer reported that when Jesus touched the eyes of the blind man, his first response was that he could see people as trees walking by. That blind man describes roughly what I see. Unfortunately I have not received a second touch, as the blind man did.

I recently decided to test just what colors I see and don't see. My assistant, Lindsay, drove me down to the Home Depot, where we looked on racks that displayed hundreds of variations of color. She must have grabbed about forty for me to identify. I had not realized before reading a book on color that there are 1 million shades of color. There were no great surprises except for the fact of how little color variations I can detect. I can see white and black. I can see red in a number of its manifestations and tints. Green is almost completely gone except that I detect either blue or green in certain dark colors. I cannot separate the dark blue from the green. I had better luck with blue, light blue especially. I can see the light blue of the sky. There is a broad countertop in a restaurant that I frequent that is light blue, and I feast my eyes observing it. I can detect tan, but not brown apparently. Although I cannot see yellow on a flat surface, I can see my lighted globe, the color of which is yellow.

The psychologist Frank H. Mahnke indicates that I might not be so bad off. He found that people confined to environments of very bright colors can be affected negatively and become subdued and dull. People in environments that are subdued become withdrawn and restless. He recommends the golden mean that would include some but not excessive variety of colors.

John Ruskin pointed out that even sighted people often do not really see. Like Wordsworth, Ruskin believed that "Little we see in nature that is ours." In describing the *Apollo and the Pythian*, Ruskin states that either viewers do not look accurately at the sky, or remember the exact shades and tones that occasionally appear in the sky. Viewers of Turner's paintings thus accuse them of being unrealistic. If one of the frames of Turner's paintings would suddenly be juxtaposed against the sky, the colors viewers would see would be even stranger and more intense at times than what Turner depicts on the canvas. We see this phenomenon in grade school too. Ask children to color the trunks of trees. The children would usually pick brown. How many trunks of trees are actually brown? Perhaps I can compensate for my visual inability to see many shades of color by noticing exactly what colors I do see. I increase my focus on a scene by asking myself, "If I were to paint this landscape around me, exactly what colors and techniques would I use?"

Walter Pater argues that experience itself, not the result of experience, is success in life, and that not to perceive each moment's experience vividly is failure in life. "Every moment some form grows perfect in hand or face; some tone on the hills or the sea is the choicer than the rest; some mood of passion or insight or intellectual excitement is irresistibly real and attractive to us,—for that moment only. Not the fruit of experience, but experience itself, is the end. A counted number of pulses only is given to us of a variegated, dramatic life. How may we see in them all that is to be seen in them by the finest senses? How shall we pass most swiftly from point to point, and be present always at the focus where the greatest number of vital forces unite in their purest energy?"

I can recall two times when I experienced the color and beauty of nature vividly. One day at dusk, when I had good eyesight, my aunt was driving me along the shore of Lake Champlain. Suddenly I said, "Aunt Helen, stop the car!" The air, lake, trees, and mountains had morphed into something strangely beautiful. I recall driving by Racquet Lake in the Adirondacks. Sometimes the view of the lake is unexceptional. At other times it displays startling beauty. At such moments my reaction has been, in the words of Emily Dickenson, "zero at the bone."

I guess the thought that some therapy might restore my vision would really excite me. Perhaps the hope that there might be some treatment for age-related macular degeneration could help sustain me; so I don't say, "nevermore." With the growing awareness of the disappearance of my color vision, I need to assess how this loss has affected my thinking and my emotional life and all my sensibilities. Writing about this loss forces me to do the thinking that I have not brought myself around to.

Part II: The Psychological Dimensions of Color

Things are not always what they seem. Often the process of education is to move beyond naïve realism. The sun seems to move around the earth. We have no awareness that we are whirling about on the globe at a fantastic speed. Light seems to be white until we see a rainbow or a prism and realize that white light is a mixture of colors, mainly red, blue, and yellow.

One fact about color has always bothered me. I learned that the color green is not really part of trees and grass. Rather it's the colors thrown off by trees and grass. The trees absorb *red* and throw off yellow and blue, or green. Things are not what they seem! I'd like to think that the green in the leaves of the tree and the hills and the grasslands is an essential part of their identity, not just some spectrum of the color they have thrown off. Not only is the color we see not of the essence of an object, but our perception of color is not color itself. Perhaps Marvel was accurate in calling the green of the park "a green thought in a green shade." The retina is composed of 120 million rods and 6 million cones. The images that the rods and cones receive are translated into electrical impulses which are sent to the brain through the optic nerve. Whoa! The brain is not getting any color, it is simply getting an electrical charge. It sounds so very mechanical! How can I grab hold of the real green or the real red? Once as a child I viewed some cans of paint. How wonderful! The green paint and the red paint and the blue paint appeared to be some kind of ultimate, like Plato's chair image. Now I am told that the only thing I am getting is a piece of electricity. I long not only to receive electrical impulses of beauty, but to become part of that beauty, whatever that means. C.S. Lewis opines that all poets thirst after not the perception of beauty, but becoming a part of beauty itself.

Of course, scientists destroy many of our illusions. We don't really see an object; we simply see the light that the object sends forth. We don't really feel a solid object; we feel a hunk of electricity. That which is solid is not really so, they say. As I read it, a desk is just a heap of electricity. It might even be strings of electricity constantly wriggling. What happened to the solid earth?

Even more disturbing to me is the thought that time is not really sequential. I've always been disturbed by the phrase in the gospel song "and time shall be no more." My assistant tells me that in the book of Revelation an angel rolls up the sea like a scroll and repeats the statement that time is to be no more. I've always been bothered by prophets and psychics who profess to see into the future. It bothers me that theologians say that God knows the future. How can God know the future if it hasn't happened? I know that Armenians say that foreknowledge does not mean predestination. I still don't like the idea of God's foreknowledge. It is beyond my comprehension why Art Bell and George Noorey, hosts of Coast to Coast AM, desire to travel to the past and to the future. I am one with Alexander Pope, who states, "Oh blindness to the future! kindly giv'n."

When my grandfather was doing carpentry in Burlington, Vermont, a psychic kept approaching him with the offer to foretell what would happen in his life. He would not listen to her, but she insisted on saying, "You will face a great tragedy in your life." When his son, my father, drowned at age twenty eight, my grandfather wondered if the psychic had actually seen the future.

Now I have tried to wrap my mind around Einstein's theory of relativity. It tires my brain to try to understand it, and I waver between thinking that time is totally relevant or simply relevant to the particular observer. I hope the latter is the case. I wonder, if God is the observer, then the events are not relevant, but absolute in time. Since I'm on this roll, I have concluded that the bottom line of the universe, so far as mankind goes, is mystery. If atheists cannot explain where the world came from, theists can't understand where God came from. One day at Fort Myer in Virginia, I was declared Soldier of the Day and given the whole day off to do whatever I liked. I could go to the PX or the commissary or walk along the streets. Instead I chose to take myself to the parade ground and write letters in the bleachers. Out of the corner of my eye, I observed an eight-year-old boy approaching. I do not know why he was not in school or what he was doing wandering around the parade grounds by himself. Upon seeing me turn around to observe him, he, without any introductory greeting, asked the most impossible question anyone can ask, "Where did God come from?" Now I may have been Soldier of the Day, but even if I were Solomon in all his wisdom and glory, I couldn't have answered that question. Bishop Berkeley removes us even farther from the physical world, stating that nothing is real but thoughts about reality. Of course, Dr. Johnson kicked a stone to refute this abstract notion.

Even more strange than the fact that color is transmitted from the eye to the brain by electrical impulses is the fact that color remains in the mind without any impulses at all. We can remember color. Once in a while we even dream in color. How can the mind remember color? Although I cannot see green trees and green grass, I can remember mowing green grass and pulling green weeds and painting my uncle's row boats with delicious green paint. My assistant points out to me that at least I have the memory of colors: something that people who are born blind lack. It seems to me that in childhood, colors are especially vibrant and important. I can recall the orange front of a sweater my parents gave me, making me look like a robin in spring. In Upstate New York, robins are one of the few birds that we could see. Bird watching books that talked of scarlet tanagers and blue jays presented a world that was tantalizingly removed from us hearty souls in the North Country. The red of Christmas against the white snow and black branches portrayed life and joy in a dead world. How green was spring grass once the snow covering the ground has melted. I remember the first Northern Lights that I witnessed. Even the story about the pot of gold at the end of the rainbow seemed remotely possible. After days of clouds of March and April, the light blue of the sky was a treasure to behold.

Some other memories come back to me. I was fascinated with coloring Easter eggs. With the little tablet dropped into hot water, a magic potion was created, into which one would dip the plain white egg. Baptized, it came out a purple or blue or fresh green. I especially liked the light green and the light blue ones. I was introduced to that wonderful thing called the Kaleidoscope and spent hours watching those colored bits of glass with the help of mirrors, forming snowflakes of colored design. And then, I would look at my bag of marbles and delight in the swirls of colors that are embedded in those smooth glass beads. How could the cleverness of man create those swirls of varied colors embedded in this solid orb? Here in my hand, I could hold substance more beautiful than a topaz or emerald or diamond. No modern artist can surpass the explosion of colors which was the Sandy Creek County Fair. Tents, merry-go-rounds, clowns, hot dog stands, ring tosses, and fireworks formed the wonderful mélange of color. I remember the colors that I can no longer see. How is it that the mind can create colors even when there is no stimulus to produce these colors? Are colors an idea?

Part III: Spiritual or Metaphysical Aspects of Color

Reading Ruskin's thoughts on color has made me consider the relation of the physical world of light and color to the abstract world of the spirit. Like Ruskin, I was reared on sermons that apply tropological thinking of the physical world to the spiritual world. How many sermons have I heard comparing the deliverance of the Israelites from Egypt to the deliverance of the individual from the realm of worldliness and sin? The New Testament itself records the address of Jesus to the Samaritan woman at Jacob's well, comparing the water of that well with the life-giving spirit that He offers. In his pontifical way, Ruskin pronounces that color in the world is the only evidence of God's love for man. I assume Ruskin was thinking of the appearance of the rainbow that supposedly is evidence from God that the world will never be destroyed again by flood. I believe what's always intrigued me about Ruskin is that he sees, like Wordsworth, the natural world as emblematic and analogous to the world of ideas. Just this morning it occurred to me that just as there are three persons in the Trinity, there are three primary colors. These colors are united in the white light that permeates the universe. Perhaps this analogy proves nothing, but it is thought provoking. It certainly is a better analogy than St. Patrick's, who considered the three leaf clover as also illustrating the Trinity.

Ruskin paid special attention to red, a color which is apparently always distinguishable, even by people who are color blind. The red of the sun is observed only when it passes through the atmosphere, especially the atmosphere marked by haze or clouds. Only when God's light enters the earth's atmosphere does the red appear. God's presence similarly only manifests itself as love for mankind as it enters the affairs of human life. Ruskin then proceeds to identify red as the color of life, as in blood. Since blood is shed, it is also the color of sacrifice. In many religions of the world, the gods are approached only through the shedding of blood. Christians interpret the shedding of the sacrificial blood of animals as a type of Christ's shedding of blood on Calvary. My own Christian belief is that the death of Christ on Calvary is emblematic of the choice that the Trinity makes to participate in man's suffering, and all people's alienation and suffering throughout all ages. Frankly I'd never thought of color as evidence of love, but I like the idea anyway.

From reading Ruskin by day, I listen to Coast to Coast AM by night. I'm sure the more rational of my readers will think that I am terribly irrational to do so. Nevertheless, I must argue that along with tons of nonsense, Coast to Coast AM explores ideas and facts that the established media and educational community dare not touch. Along with UFOs, ghosts, out-of-body experiences, and prophecies, the program will also invite leading scholars and scientists to present their ideas. One nameless scientist on the program seemed to be in sync with Ruskin. This scientist believes that there is more than symbolic relationship between light in the universe and the power and presence of the Almighty in His creation. There is an absolute quality, he noted, about light. Nothing is faster than light. Light permeates the universe and has done so ever since the Big Bang thirteen and a half billion years ago.

Light exists even though the human eye cannot perceive it; for the spectrum of light goes both below human perception in ultra violet light and above the spectrum that the eye can see in X-Rays. All objects emit light and can be called, in some sense, light itself. Many religions worship the sun or what the sun symbolizes. In Kenya, before the arrival of Christianity, the natives worshipped the sun, and yet not the sun itself, but something behind the sun. Zoroastrians include light at the center of their worship. Every temple is centered on a huge fire. In Buddhism all beings are said to posses a spark of inner light. Jewish mystics speak of the spark of God. Krishna, Buddha, Allah, as well as Judaism and Christianity, all speak of God as light. The Psalmist asked, "Where can we flee from God's presence? Even in the depths of Sheol, He is there," in the same way that light is everywhere. There's nowhere that light images are used so extensively as in the New Testament. God is portrayed as light, in whom there is no shadow of turning. Jesus is the light that lighteth every man that comes into the world. We are enjoined to walk in the light. We are warned against letting the light in us become darkness because then how great that darkness will be. After all, there are black holes which swallow light. What about people that are totally blind? Yet, even they can feel the warmth of light. In some way the light in color that sighted people observe can be reflected through words and ideas to those that are totally blind. People like me are fortunate enough to see some color, in any case, and much light.

I was intrigued when George Noorey explained how he kept himself from the negative subjects he often deals with on Coast to Coast. Whether ghosts and demons and reptilians are real or not, thoughts of these can pollute the mind. Even dwelling on them in one's thoughts can have a negative impact. He stated that at night when he retires, mentally he wraps himself in light. I think I know this much, that in this dark world, our primary obligation is to not only observe ourselves faithfully and honestly, but to follow the inner light that the Quakers talked about. It is not enough to discover truth simply by the light of intellect since truth is not some mathematical game of the mind. It is important to respond to what we do know is right and true, step by step. I also believe, with Neo-Platonists, that physical beauty can be a stepping stone to higher beauty. And how is beauty received but through light and color? Cardinal Newman put it well in his poem "Lead, Kindly Light." He wrote, "I do not ask to see the distant scene, one step enough for me."

Chapter Six:

Wilt Thou be Healed?

Yesterday, as I was walking with my mobility cane through the student center to a discussion group, a young man accosted me, asking me if anyone had ever prayed for my healing. I said yes. I could have detailed to him the occasions. One time in the Atlanta Greyhound Bus Terminal the man I had ridden with from Columbus, Ohio, placed his hands on my shoulder and prayed for a miracle. Then at a religious healing service, a dear man came over, put his arms around my shoulder, and asked if I would go forward to be healed. After I gave a lecture on Matthew Arnold in my British literature class, a young man hugged me and prayed that my sight would be restored. Recently as I walked down Broadway past the courthouse, a sidewalk preacher seeing me pass by with a mobility cane called out to the Almighty, saying, "Jesus heal this blind man." A young lady I meet frequently at the bus stop inquired as to what church I attended. She wanted to know if it was "a healing church." What she meant by that question exactly, I don't know, but I suspect she wanted to know if it was a church emphasized divine healing and maybe promised it to all.

I later found out through reading that other blind people had become targets of would-be-healers. Georgina Kleege records in her book *Sight Unseen* that she was approached in an airplane terminal by a lady who claimed to be "Catholic Mother of the Year in Ohio," and asked permission to pray for her as crowds milled around the terminal. John Hull in his book *Touching the Rock* mentions being approached by a fervent healer who volunteered to come to Hull's house and pray for him. This prayer warrior returned to find out that Hull was not healed. The prayer warrior was not to be put off. He persisted, "If you will carry this New Testament around with you for two weeks in obedience to God, then you will be healed." It would not surprise me if most blind people do not encounter the same offers for prayer.

I have no idea who my latest prayer warrior was. I assume he was a student at the university, probably a freshman. My bet is that he didn't know who I was. He seemed not to be aware or care that I was professor emeritus at the university. He did not even ask my name or introduce himself. He surmised, accurately, that I was visually handicapped because I was walking with the mobility cane. Oh the mobility cane. It lets everyone know within hailing distance that the owner is visually handicapped. Most times the user is the only one within ten miles with a white cane. How can someone avoid being noticed with that symbol in one's hand? Of course the other side of the coin is one wants people to notice that one is handicapped. You can't have one without the other. You can't want people to see that you are blind and on the other hand not notice you as a special case. You are a walking spectacle. I can sympathize with a sentiment from Bob Dylan's song that describes a person as a "walking antique." Because of her strange physiognomy and unusual dress, the poet Edith Sitwell was described as "a high altar on the move." So I proclaimed to all in the hallway yesterday that

I was visually handicapped. This young man saw that I was not whole and, stirred by religious fervor or humane feelings or both, moved himself to action. It certainly is a strange place to have a prayer meeting, in the middle of the hallway when people are streaming by. But as the old spiritual says, "It's me, O Lord, standing in the need of prayer." When Doctor Samuel Johnson heard the criticism of the poet Kit Smart, namely that the poet would drop down on his knees on any occasion to pray, Johnson responded, "I don't know whether it's more irrational to drop down on your knees at unusual occasions to pray than it is not to pray at all."

Although I told the student I had already been prayed for, he persisted with the question, "Would you permit me to pray for you?"

"That would be fine," I agreed. Although the situation was rather odd, I was not about to treat his offer sarcastically. Soon enough life will teach him to trim his fervor, and to dampen his urge to offer help to his neighbor.

Before saying the prayer, the healer opened up the Bible to Isaiah and read, "He was wounded for our transgressions, and by his stripes we are healed." Then he proceeded to pray a short formulaic prayer, lacking in rhetorical flourish or emotional intensity. I will say that the passersby did not stand around to gawk. We opened our eyes, and he asked, "How do you feel?" I could have said, in the words of the popular song, "I woke up this morning feeling fine, I woke up with heaven on my mind." However, I did not answer his question, since I felt that he probably wanted me to say, "I felt a surge of healing power flow through my body, and lo! I can now see." Had my eyes been restored, there probably would have been a media event rivaling that of John Howard Griffin's, whose sight was suddenly restored after ten years of blindness. He was besieged by reporters and forced to hide himself in a monastery until the storm passed.

Now I thanked the young man for his concern. I did not want to hurt this young man's feelings or his faith. The worst thing in the world that I could have done would have been to utter some wise crack. On the other hand, I wanted to correct his thinking that anyone who asks for healing would automatically be healed. He said, "Well the promise is in the bible."

To which I replied, "Also in the bible is Saint Paul's statement that 'Though he asked for the thorn to be removed from his flesh, God did not grant his request, but God did say 'My grace is sufficient for you.'"

"I didn't know that was in the Bible," said this budding theologian. Rather than continue to discuss a theological debate in the hallway, and since I was already late for my meeting, I invited him to stop by my office. Now I did forget to tell him who I was, so perhaps I should not expect him to stop by. Somehow, I doubt that he would have anyway. Should he drop by, I probably would have argued my own position, and not only argued my position, but dialogued with him about the issue. If he had dropped by, I would have said, "Come on and sit down, Dale. Have you had classes in this building before?"

He might have replied, "Yes. I took freshman composition in room 202."

I would then ask, "Dale, what is your major?"

He would have responded, "I am an accounting major."

I then would ask, "Who has informed your opinion of divine healing?"

He would say, "Reverend Skywatch at the Heavenly Rainbow Church recently preached a series of sermons on the subject."

On receiving this information, I would have said, "Well, Dale, I don't expect everyone to agree with me, but I have some thoughts on divine healing that I'd like to share with you and see what you think. First, I'd like to say that I believe in the possibility of divine healing—if not in this life, in the life to come. We are all going to die unless there is some kind of rapture or something. No one is given the gift of eternal life and health in this world. After all, scripture says the last enemy to be conquered is death itself. And Dale, I don't look at the real purpose of scripture to be that we shall live a wealthy, healthy, happy, fulfilled life on this earth. I don't really believe in the prosperity gospel. However, I do believe that following the principles set forth in the scriptures tends to lead to a happy and healthy life. Still, everyone is subjected to disappointment, illness, and eventually death. Now, since I have not been healed of my visual handicap or my arthritic knee, I have experienced a healing of sorts recently. When the urologist discovered that I was retaining much urine and blood, he asked me to monitor my condition carefully. I asked the urologist, 'Do you think I might have cancer?' The urologist responded, 'Yes. That's one of the options.' I remember sitting for devotions and saying in an unimpassioned way, 'God, you can heal me if you will.' Now whether it was a divine intimation or my imagination, I was surprised to feel that everything would be okay. It turned out that I did not have cancer, and, after an operation on my bladder and prostate, the doctor said excitedly, 'Your recovery is miraculous.' So you see, Dale, I am not some intellectual cynic." As often happens while I was talking about my medical problem, one of my colleagues would have dropped into my office at this juncture to remind me that recovering from an operation is an easy thing in comparison to having one's eyesight restored. "Mike," I would have said, "Just because I believe that healing occurs sometimes does not mean that I believe it occurs at all times." That response would have quieted

Mike down. "So now, Dale, don't you believe that too much emphasis on healing is a distortion of the gospel?"

Dale would have answered, "Well if more people got healed, God would be glorified, and more people would be saved."

"You've got a point there. I don't understand, Dale, why God doesn't heal more people. I have seen cases of divine healing. My ten-year-old brother as far as I can tell was healed from diabetes one, and although diabetes one never returned, he did contract diabetes two. There is a senior pastor from my church who traveled with a group to Europe and Palestine. According to all thirty on the trip, Reverend Joe Morgan came down with such an occurrence of arthritis that he decided to return to the United States before completing the trip. While they were at the river Jordan, he felt led to be baptized there in front of the group. After the baptism, he immediately lost all traces of arthritis and ran all over Europe. Until his death, he had no reoccurrence of his arthritis. On the other hand, Dale, I have seen all kinds of suffering and deserving people who were fervently prayed for and who were not healed."

"They probably didn't have enough faith," Dale would have said. "If you have faith the size of a mustard seed, you can ask what you will, and it will be done unto you."

"Well Dale, I remind you of what I said before that Saint Paul asked for the thorn to be removed from his flesh, but it wasn't removed, was it? Dale, I don't understand why some people are healed and some are not healed, but if we follow the scripture, we will pray for healing as we are commanded to do. I really don't believe that we are supposed to muster up some sort of high-powered belief that we shall be healed in order that healing will take place. I know you don't like the kind of prayer that I grew up with: God please heal me *if* it be your will. I taught with a man named J.A. Felter. He recounted that in a terrible accident, his wife was critically injured. He prayed desperately that she live. His prayer was answered, supposedly. She did live, but she was almost a vegetable that had to be pushed around in a wheelchair. The old saints that I grew up around believed that in prayer you could receive a mystical leading as to whether the healing was in God's will or not. They used to use another term that I no longer hear. They "prayed through" an issue, meaning whatever God chose to do or not do, their prayer had been heard or answered. What do you think of that, Dale?"

Backing down, Dale would have said, "I agree with most of what you said."

"You don't have to agree with me, Dale, and neither does the reader of this book. I am not preaching, I'm just telling you what I think. There you have it. I am a mystic believer of sorts. I am okay with the label. Whether you approve my position or not, so be it. I have a final word for you, Dale: come in any time, and we'll go for coffee. Again, I appreciate your concern and your faith and your willingness to listen to me, and your willingness to disagree with me too. You're welcome to stop me anytime in any place and say a prayer for me because I'm standing in the need of prayer and wisdom." About this time, Dale would have grown restless. As often seems the case, the more I win an argument, the less my opponent wants to hear it, and so Dale would have hastily retreated from the office, and I would have reproached myself for having talked too much, and for being so clever that my listener was either cowed into silence, or, out of courtesy, chose to remain somewhat mute. I just cannot allow silence to reign, and if my visitor doesn't talk, I must rush in with words. I could have gone on and talked about the fact that virtually all Christian denominations believe in healing, and I had recently read *Science and Health with Keys to the Scripture*, in which Mary

Baker Eddy believes that sickness and evil are identical. Even though the book has many beautiful passages, I could not agree totally with the author.

I am not alone in having some ideas on the subject of divine healing, although it has not been a major preoccupation of mine. I am aware that virtually all Christian traditions professed to believe in divine healing, and that certain groups like Christian Scientists and Charismatics emphasize that belief.

I think that possibly a person may be led to pray for healing. Some people, like me, feel that they should not ask for healing. I have never been able to figure out why some are given divine healing and some are not. After the man who urged me to go forward in the church service for healing saw me the next day, he said, "I'm very sorry that you were not healed."

I responded, "I'm doing very well with my limited eyesight and have not felt led to ask for healing." Our dialogue might have covered more subjects than divine healing, and I am willing to be taught by anybody, young or old, with a person with similar views or with a person with drastically different views.

Chapter Seven:

I Get By With a Little Help from My Friends

It's an ill wind that does not blow someone some good, goes the saying. One of the surprising benefits of having macular degeneration is the introduction into my life of a number of helpers. I suppose if I were married, I could rely on my wife, at least partly, to aid me in the many tasks of survival. Not having a wife, I have had to rely on others. Now I am fiercely independent. For example, I have a hard time living in anyone else's home, even longer than several days. I am reluctant to impose on others for rides or help in reading or shopping. I have tried not to bother those around me by asking for help. If I can figure out a way to handle my own affairs, I try to do so. Fortunately many of my friends volunteer to drive me to a party or take me home from an evening function at school since the bus around the campus does not run after 6:00 PM. Occasionally I even ask for a ride, but I do so sparingly. Although I cannot drive, I have two feet. In fact I look on walking to shop or to eat as an opportunity for exercise. How much better it is to walk when you have a practical goal in mind than simply to walk on a treadmill or walk around the block! I am fortunate also to have access to bus routes. While North Park, San Diego, may not be the most elegant place to live, it is certainly the most convenient for a bus rider. Four different bus routes are situated near my home. During the day, the Number 7 bus runs every fifteen minutes to the center of the city. Then there are taxis. If I am tempted to think of taxis as an extravagance, I have only to remind myself how expensive it is to keep a car by feeding it gasoline and seeing that it is in working order.

To pay my bills and help in my teaching and writing, I have a bevy of young people whom I pay small sums. Dr. Johnson made it a point to be friends with young people, since many of his contemporaries, having grown old, were dying off. I have acquired a number of delightful young people to help me with clerical tasks. Dwight and Ted stop by the house occasionally. We go through bills and papers. Ted goes with me to the grocery store since it is hard to pick out what I need in the blur of items that crowd the aisles. Ted had been one of my English majors when I was sighted. On running into each other on a bus, he asked if I needed any help. I was fortunate enough to find that he had some time available to read to me and to help me sort out papers, and Dwight, who is absolutely trustworthy, helps me pay bills and organize papers during income tax time. He is also handy in keeping my electric and electronic items working correctly. Recently he honored me by asking me to read a poem at his wedding. While I was still teaching full-time at the university, the school allowed me four hours a week of student help. After they became aware that I was visually handicapped, they allowed me much more student help. The names of these wonderful students flash into mind— Matt Demangos, Rachel Contraros, and David Anthony. After I retired in the year 2000, the school was generous enough to offer me part-time use of an office. The first year of retirement, I taught a Shakespeare class. I began hiring students on my own to help me with that class and then later with a few directed studies. They also helped me compose books on the computer. Now I confess, to my great shame, that throughout my entire teaching career I was without the ability to type. My handwriting was very clear, and I had office secretaries who unfailingly typed up my tests and worksheets. I don't regret being without the ability to type my doctoral thesis, since I could spend all my time doing the research and the actual writing without being concerned with margins and spacing and neatness that was required for both seminar papers and my doctoral dissertation. A student typed my doctoral dissertation, but the week before I was to leave to defend it, she became ill. I left, then, on the train to Washington, D.C. with a number of pages that needed to be corrected. The horse was really in the ditch. In this crisis, I called Mrs. Behrens, a woman who lived in College Park, Maryland, and who had typed my seminar papers for the University of Maryland. In a panic, I called her explaining my situation. Although she was swamped with other papers, she agreed to make the corrections. I should add that in those days, we relied on typewriters, carbon paper, and onionskin duplicates.

In my last years of teaching, the school pressured all faculty to become computer competent. One day I walked into my office to discover a large, ugly computer sitting on my desk, even though I hadn't asked for the monstrosity. Trying to avoid being dragged into the computer age, I covered the screen with a large sign which read, "Trojan Horse." For inside my bastion of Luddism, they had inserted this modern invention, an endeavor to force my use of it. I gradually realized that I must come into the computer age, even though I was dragged thrashing and screaming into it. I was not only pressured to learn how to type because a voice-activated system for computers still has too many bugs in it, I was forced to begin typing on the computer itself.

As I mentioned earlier, clouds tend to have silver linings. The school provided me with a voice-activated program. It taught me how to type because it let me know immediately when I hit the wrong key. Thanks be to computers. I now use typing along with dictation as the means of composing my writing. If I try to write with a pen, I make an awful mess since I tend to write over what I have already written. Along with most every other writer, I know that computers make revision easy.

Now it is important for my assistants to have computer skills. There followed a number of wonderful students who not only brightened my office themselves, but attracted their other college friends into the office. Jon Munn, a philosophy major who minored in literature, would come into the office with his baseball cap turned backwards, which covering most of his red hair. Often we would depart from the work at hand to discuss ideas. After Jon Munn I had a succession of young helpers. Rachel Mournian, her son Matthew, not a student, Marilyn Hydra, Eileen Chen, Brook Pate, Dominic Tarantino, and Lindsay Preston all brought life and faithful work into my office. I did learn not to have three students working on the same computer.

One day I met a student in the hallway. She greeted me with a quotation from a Shakespeare play, given in a British dialect, "The quality of mercy is not strained/ It droppeth as the gentle rain from heaven/ Upon the earth beneath it is twice blessed/ Blesseth him that gives and him that takes." She asked me if I liked Shakespeare. She followed me into my office, informing me that she was a student in a class where I had given a guest lecture. She told me about the Shakespeare club she had formed in high school and went on to brag about several of her literature teachers, informing me that they had broadened her literary tastes to include many other writers other than Shakespeare. I am not sure just how she discovered in what state of confusion I was with my computer. It does not take Morgan Cooper long to discover the lay of the land, and she saw that I was in need of some efficient help. She soon discovered that my problem lay in having several assistants, and she decided to replace them when they left with one assistant—herself. I, of course, realized that many cooks spoil the broth. There was no need of a radio or stereo in my office, since Morgan sang snatches from musicals whenever the opportunity offered itself. Morgan was more than just a typist or organizer; she became an on-location critic and editor and cheerleader. The success of my writing became her goal. She had faith that what I was composing was worthwhile.

Eventually Morgan graduated and went to Europe. But she would not leave before finding me a replacement that suited her standards. After proposing several, she settled on one of her friends whom she had made in the literature classes, April Anderson. She brought April in one afternoon to learn the ropes, and soon April was performing the same tasks as was Morgan, though without the Shakespeare quotations and without the opera. April was a writing major, and Morgan realized that she possessed editorial skills that most students lack. It was through April that we started a small writer's group that met several times at my condominium.

I have mentioned that I rely heavily on public transportation to get around. Public transportation is perfectly adequate for traveling to my athletic club and my office and my church. But when I travel to Upstate New York to visit relatives and attend the annual Tamarack Writers Conference, it is inadequate. How could I travel from Syracuse, New York, where I get off the airplane, to Big Moose Lake in the Adirondacks? There are no trains, no planes, and no buses that make that journey. Fortunately I had a brother, Steve, who lived forty miles from the writers conference. Like me, he was retired and so was able to chauffer me around the state. He was more than willing to perform this duty, but I helped with the car expenses, and this arrangement aided him, too. It was a symbiotic relationship. I might add that my brother was a good salesman for my book *Upstarts in Upstate*. In fact, when I visit my other brother and sisters, they provide wheels for my convenience. It has probably helped my attitude in accepting the loss of being able to drive that I did not own a car until I was in my late twenties. I spent most of my money on going to school. So it was that I was used to walking and taking a bus and hitching a ride with others. Of course, I no longer hitchhike as I did when I was much younger. I would doubt if an aging man would get many rides. Furthermore, hitchhiking has become too dangerous for both the hitchhiker and the driver who picks up the hitchhiker. The law of life is change, and the only response that is essential for us is to be flexible and change with the change. I have been reading the book *Tuesdays with Morrie*. My handicap is trivial beside his ALS disease. He had to learn to accept help, even in elementary bodily functions. How fortunate am I compared to this man. And yet the book inspires us readers because he accepted his dependency on others with a grace that gave a certain dignity to what would be considered demeaning tasks. Perhaps his greatest fear was, as he put it, that someone would have to wipe his bottom. But eventually, he accepted even that necessity. It surely is more blessed to give help to others than to receive it for oneself. But, the latter is still possible to accept with resignation.

I have often observed that to grow old gracefully is the final gift one can give to those who surround him or her. I have known those who grew old gracefully and those who grew old with bitterness. It is easy, I know, to pontificate on what a person should do who is both old and ill. The test will come, perhaps, to me. If I not only add years to my life and add a visual handicap to my ability, but also serious illness and pain to my lot, I hope that I will remember my own preachments, and that I will inspire those around me with cheerfulness and philosophical acceptance. Perhaps I will give the lie to my own teaching.

CHAPTER EIGHT:

Etiquette for the World of Blindness

Like most children, Lewis Carroll's Alice is eager to have clear rules of conduct and limits to behavior. In Wonderland she is constantly being frustrated by the unexpected, the strange, and the irrational. Alice is no stranger to the game of croquet, but in Wonderland the rules of croquet do not obtain. As strange as the appearance and disappearance of the Cheshire cat, so the set up of Wonderland croquet baffles this well-intentioned young lady. All her expectations are thwarted. The Queen, who referees the game, behaves in a completely arbitrary fashion. Only her vanity remains constant. Her sole response to others is to order their heads to be lopped off.

Alice finds the croquet ground to be in utter confusion. All the arches are composed of soldiers standing upside down. The balls are hedgehogs rolled up, and for mallets, players are to use flamingo heads. The problem is that the soldiers wander around the playing field, the hedgehogs unroll themselves at will, and the flamingos are more intent on examining Alice's face than in hitting the hedgehog. Now Alice has an ear in which to voice her complaints. I often wish I had a similar contrivance. In the sky over the croquet field appears gradually the Cheshire cat. At first only the grin appears, but later are the mouth, nose, and ears. With the onset of my visual loss, I found myself in a new playing field and have looked for new rules for this new game of life. Having no Cheshire cat for an audience, I will complain and suggest into human ears. Like the Queen's croquet game, the sighted players in this world often confuse the players who are unsighted. Through my experience of being visually handicapped, I have formulated ten rules. Here are ten situations that bother the blind, and ten rules that will help the blind cope in this game:

Commandment One. The other day, a pick-up truck turned quickly off University Avenue onto Kansas Street. Now I was walking with my mobility cane across the street. Fortunately I saw this errant vehicle and stopped as the truck swerved into where I was about to walk. I guess he either didn't see me or assumed that I could see him—a dangerous assumption since many who use the mobility cane are totally blind. A wheel chair totally ignored poor Bob's mobility cane, and the wheelchair ran over the cane, snapping it in two. The wheel chair operator did not stop. At the underpass in Old Town, a lady warned her daughter, "Watch out for the blind man." The child proceeded to walk right in front of my cane since I was turning to walk up the stairs.

Many pedestrians have no regard for the mobility cane. They will dash in front of me, depending on me to see them and to stop. Sometimes they are even running. They come into my visual field only at the last minute. If I weren't possessed with partial vision, there would have been many collisions, and I am big enough so that they would have gotten the worst out of these accidents. I would have delivered a real body blow. These moves in the game in life lead me to Commandment One: Stay out of the way of the mobility cane. Its owner may not see you, your wheelchair, or your vehicle at all. Unfortunately some sighted players seem not to be aware of what the mobility cane is. These people guess that it is a ski pole, a fishing rod, a golf club, or a regular walking stick. One fellow rider on the trolley noted that I was quite in fashion, as walking sticks were classy accouterments. From under what rock hath these people crawled?

Commandment Two. A lady at the lunch counter asked what I wanted to order. I replied, "What kind of sandwiches do you have," whereupon she waived her arm in a vague upward direction and said, "Read the menu." When I asked the position of certain things and places, like where the restroom is, a clerk may say, "Over there," pointing his hand in some direction I cannot see, or "Over here," or "Down there." One of the ladies at the DMV presented me a form to fill out. I replied, "I can't see it. I can't do it."

"Find someone to do it," she replied.

"I just did. You're the one to help me," I replied.

At Macy's I asked the clerk to direct me to the underwear section. Now I'm completely dependent on the clerk to see sizes and costs and not just to indicate vaguely where the underwear department is. It was about three in the afternoon, and I think that he was standing in need of a nap. When I asked, therefore, for the direction to the underwear department, he gave the ol' brush-off wave. Directions and information for the blind need to be spelled out, and that is Commandment Two. Bob at the Blind Center designed t-shirts on which were emblazoned, "Where is Over There?" Does the blind person carrying a mobility cane need to say every time, "I cannot see the menu on the wall. I don't know where 'Over there' means in locating the restroom"?

Commandment Three. An old college friend from the forties met me in my office and asked, "Guess who is here." Now even if I could see her, she probably has put on some pounds and wrinkles since she was a gorgeous co-ed. Since I have met in my life probably ten thousand adults of the female species, I could not identify that being standing in my office door. At the fitness center, there are a number of young women who check me in. There is Heidi, Consuelo, Teresa, Heather, Dannie, and Joelle, and they all look the same to me. When they very kindly say, "Hi Arthur," I would like to be able to say their name in response. One day I said, "Hi Consuelo."

She said, "No, I'm Heather." Well.

Walking across campus, a number of people greet me. How nice. For most of them I either say "Hi," or "Who are you?" Very few for some reason I can detect. It seems to me very discourteous for me to just say hello without recognizing the person speaking to me. But, who is it? Commandment Three: When you address a blind person, first identify who you are. It would be nice if I could see auras. It would be even nicer if I could see the people's faces themselves. When offering assistance to a blind woman, it might be a good idea to identify yourself so she does not think you are some kind of rabid rapist. When you are about to leave a conversation with any blind person, it is helpful to say that you have to do so, so that she won't be talking into vacuity to someone who is no longer there.

Commandment Four, the horrors of hors d'oeuvres. Now some people love social situations in which they can flip from one person to another. Imagine the kind of confusion that a blind person experiences, standing amidst a hundred people whom he can't identify. John M. Hull complains that when he wished to take a break and go to a bar for a drink and companionship, he is left alone, even though when he leaves a number of people greet him. "Why didn't you come and drink with me," he asked them.

They responded, "We thought you wanted to be alone." Oh how much fun it is to eat or drink alone. Commandment Four: Include the blind in your socializing at group occasions.

At events where hors d'oeuvres are served, it may be helpful to pass the blind person on to another partier. I have found that in such occasions, it is best to find a seat and sit still until other people come to talk to me. In any case, the whole purpose of hors d'oeuvres seems to be light chit-chat, and I must confess that I'm not very good at it. If someone asks me, "How are you?" I should say I'm worried about making my next mortgage payment and my brother is in the middle of a nervous break down or some such reality-based talk.

Commandment Five. Walking across campus, where there were some teenage visitors, I heard the comment, "There's a blind man." Well I'm glad she recognized the mobility cane; however, I felt a little like a leper. I felt like a rare bird that had just been spotted by a bird watcher, saying, "There's a spotted warbler!" I'm not ashamed of being blind, yet I hope that my handicap in not the entirety of how people view me. It would be nice if she had said, "There is a handsome blind man," or "Look how young that blind man is," or "That blind man looks like an interesting man to me."

When I walk into a new classroom, I try not to mention my blindness or emphasize it. After awhile, in a casual way, I will let them know that I am visually handicapped. But I don't want them to say, "A blind man has now come to teach us." Actually I don't really want to be called blind because I'm not. I like the term partially blind or visually handicapped. Please don't call me visually challenged or accuse me of having neutral vision, as these terms smack of being politically correct. Commandment Five: Try to look behind a person's handicap to see the person himself or herself.

Commandment Six. Now this is a hard one. The other day at the bus stop, a kind-hearted man asked me which bus I wanted to take. I told him that I would like to catch the

Number 2 bus. When the Number 902 bus arrived, he tried to dissuade me from boarding it, even though I can take the Number 902 bus several stops, and catch the Number 7 bus, which is even better than the Number 2 bus. His offer to help was more of a nuisance than an aid. On the other hand, I walked into a drugstore and stood among the rows and rows of products I could not see. It took some doing to track down a clerk to help me. I think it should be obvious that I could not help myself in that situation. I received an offer of a ride to a banquet. I could have easily taken the bus. When the kind man who offered failed to show up, it was too late to take the bus. His offer to help then was actually a hindrance. Commandment Six: Try to be sensitive about when to offer help and when not to.

When I am walking down the street, a companion will indicate where a curb is. If the curb is a different color than the roadway, I can figure it out myself, especially since I am expecting a curb. On the other hand, I ran into a cement seat which was the same color as the side walk. It would be very helpful if my companion had warned me that the bench was in front of me. I fell over the seat, but fortunately I did not break a bone that time. At the fitness center, the manager urged me to avail myself to the handrails as I exited the Jacuzzi, but he didn't do anything about the exercise area, which was blocked with equipment. One day, therefore, with the sun in my eyes, I tripped over a bench that blocked my path and broke my wrist.

Commandment Seven. I offered to help my friend sort out books at the San Diego Rescue Mission. Since he was a Biology teacher, he did not know how to judge literature. He was told that they didn't use handicapped people. Since my friend was right there to read the titles of the books, I failed to see how my handicap would keep me from being useful. I am sometimes invited to a wedding or a funeral, and without transportation, it is very difficult for me to attend. I was invited to a Christmas party, but the address was so complex because it was in a gated area that the taxi driver could not find it. Commandment Seven: Try to be sensitive to the abilities and disabilities of the handicapped person.

Commandment Eight. At a class where we sat in a round, my friend on the other side of the circle pointed out that I was wearing one brown sock and one black sock. Today my secretary took off a label from my shirt. One Sunday I arrived at church with my necktie half over my collar. I have been known to wear sweaters inside out and shirts buttoned unevenly. One year for Christmas, a friend gave me a necktie. Preparing for a lecture, I grabbed the necktie and wore it with my sweater. In the middle of my lecture on the poet Percy Bysshe Shelley, I heard the tune "Rudolph the Red-Nosed Reindeer." Since it was October and not December, I knew that something strange was afoot. As the lecture proceeded, I kept hearing the same song. Thinking it might be a Christmas card, I fumbled through papers on the lectern. There was no Christmas card there. The students sat as if hearing "Rudolph the Red-Nosed Reindeer" in the middle of a lecture on Shelley was normal. I couldn't think of just what to do to stop the music. At the end of the class, a sweet young girl in the front row came to the lectern and whispered, "I think it's your necktie." How was I to know that in the necktie was embedded a musical button. Every time I hit my chest, "Rudolph the Red-Nosed Reindeer" appeared.

When I have a spot on my shirt or coat or trousers, I am unfailingly told about it. Commandment Eight: Do not expect a visually handicapped person to be perfectly attired and don't give neckties embedded with music cassettes to the unwary blind man. If you do notice something that is out of kilter, tell him or her privately and let the blind person know that it's not a serious issue.

Commandment Nine. As I was riding in a car the other day, the driver said, "Will you look at that?" The answer is, "No, I will not look at it because I can't see it." On the other hand, I had a person rave at the beauties of the sunset, describing the beauty of the colors in detail, saying, "I wish you could see what I see." Commandment Eight: Let the visually handicapped person know occasionally what the scenery is but without exclaiming, "I wish you could see what I see." A vivid verbal description is always welcome.

Commandment Ten. The other day at the fitness center, I knocked over a sign telling people that the floor was wet. Walking out to the swimming pool in the path, someone had misplaced his towels on the walkway. Several years ago at a relatives' house, I almost stepped on a baby they had placed on the floor. Several weeks ago I was walking down University Avenue and happened to spot a bucket of paint sitting in the middle of the sidewalk. The painter was painting a building a few feet away. So, Commandment Ten: Keep the paths a blind man walks as free from obstacles as much as possible.

Rules for the Blind. Perhaps Alice's confusion about the croquet field also describes the uncertainty that the sighted feel when dealing with the blind. They often are not sure how to relate to blind people, and so blind people need to attempt to clear away that confusion. I would like, therefore, to suggest then rules for myself and other visually handicapped people. I believe that I have some credentials for these suggestions since I have been sighted as well as blind.

Jesus said don't try to remove a splinter in someone else's eye while at the same time you have a beam of wood in your own. Perhaps, understandably, we blind people become absorbed in our own difficulties and forget that we have a responsibility for making life easier for other people as well as asking for consideration for ourselves. What we do and how we react with other people have important consequences. In fact, if we concentrate on helping other people, we will forget some of our own problems.

Rule One. I'm not the only one involved in this social game of life. I can behave thoughtlessly to throw everyone around me into confusion or a panic. At a party, my cane stuck out and almost tripped the young lady I was with onto the ground. One day I pointed my cane to explain a direction and almost poked a bystander's eye out.

Several times I have unfolded my mobility cane and, in the process, hit the seat in front of me, thus startling the fat lady across the aisle. Dogs sometimes are frightened by the mobility cane, thinking that I am holding it to hit them. Rule One: As much as is possible, make your presence and your attitude helpful to other people. Manners, after all, consist of doing unto others as you would have them do unto you.

Rule Two. One night at dinner at a fancy restaurant, I knocked over a water glass, an act that made the table wet and soaked several dresses and trousers. Since I knew that I couldn't see it, I should have moved my silverware and reached for my glass carefully. My friend is always moving some of my food in the middle of the plate, since I tend to spill lettuce leaves and slices of bread onto the table cloth. Rule Two: Since I know that I am blind, I need to be careful in moving objects about my plate and on the table. I have been known to place wrapped butter packets in my mouth. I also, horrors, in feeling for food in a cafeteria line, have stuck my fingers into salad dressing and cake icing. Perhaps I poisoned several with this careless behavior. I notice that when I take doughnuts to the California Council for the Blind, some of my fellow blind people paw over the doughnuts instead of simply taking the first one their hands touch. Who wants to eat a doughnut that has been pawed by twenty different hungry visually handicapped creatures? One lady must have a chocolate doughnut. Nothing else will do. Another lady insisted that an apple fritter had too many calories for her.

Rule Three. I have a friend who volunteers to drive me to church. I have a neighbor who will take me to any doctor appointment. My sisters volunteered to fly to San Diego to help me after an operation that involved a one-day visit to the hospital. Now while I appreciate these offers, I can survive by taking the bus and occasionally hiring my assistant to stay overnight when I return from the operation. There is no reason I can't rely occasionally on taxis rather than inconveniencing a friend. After all, I am saving lots of money by not owning a car. Rule Three: Don't call for help when you do not need it.

On the other hand, when help is really needed, I have to accept it graciously. After all, no man is an island. Even when someone offers help that is not wanted, I should be gracious in thanking the well-intentioned person. One day, a lady grabbed my arm to steer me across the street. The beeper let me know that I could walk, and I can see the markers for the crosswalk. Still I did not pull away from her, and I thanked her. At airports, assistance is provided for me by way of a wheelchair. I should not insist on walking behind the wheelchair even though I am able to do it. Even though I could ask for assistance at the supermarket, I can pay an assistant to help me shop rather than relying on one of the busy workers there at the market.

Rule Four. It is natural to talk about one's own problems. "May I show you my operation," does not really excite general interest in whoever is going to see it, especially if it is on an indelicate place on the body. The temptation is to talk about one's own problems, be it blindness or whatever. I am thinking now of a young man who is blind and friendly, but, so far as I can tell, has shown not one iota of interest in any person other than himself. Rule Four: Focus one's attention on other people's concerns instead of on one's visual handicap. In a sense, everyone is disabled. As the saying goes, "I complained because I had no shoes till I met a man who has no feet." I saw an ad in a newspaper that reflected the spirit of this rule. It read, "He who dries another's tears will never weep alone. He who calms his brother's fears need never be afraid."

Rule Five. I have seen totally blind people move in a most ungainly fashion. Alex at the Blind Center thrashes about as he walks. Anyone who is in the hallway must dodge his flailing arms and legs. Other totally blind people stick their mobility cane out in awkward and jerky fashions. Sometimes totally blind people have not learned to face the person who is talking to them and respond with appropriate facial gestures. Sometimes blind people are not aware of ticks or other nervous reactions that are not pleasing to the onlooker. I know that even totally blind people can appear and act in a gracious fashion. My Braille instructor, Evelyn, is an excellent example of such appearance and behavior. Rule Five: The totally blind person should seek instruction and help so that his looks and behavior should be more socially acceptable.

Rule Six. When I was young I met several blind people who frightened me with their distance and seriousness. I resolved when I became partially blind that I would keep a sense of humor, smile a lot, and try to be outgoing and friendly. I am not sure that I have kept that vow very carefully, but I am trying. Even before becoming visually handicapped, I sometimes had difficulty in initiating a conversation. It seemed better to wait until others did so. Then I could show my friendliness and humor.

My mother had a number of sayings that have stuck with me. One by Edwin Markham is applicable at this juncture:

> He drew a circle that shut me out
> Heretic, rebel, a thing to flout
> But love and I had the wit to win:
> We drew a circle that took him in.

Rule Six: Attempt to portray a friendly, optimistic, and cheerful demeanor. I can add a little rhyme by Ella Wheeler Wilcox, "Laugh, and the world laughs with you; weep, and you weep alone."

Rule Seven. When I lost my visual acuity, I looked for mechanical means to help me read and write. Almost accidentally I stumbled upon a Kurzweil machine called the Reading Edge, which Xerox donated to the school for my benefit. Since that time I have learned that there are a number of machines, services, and helps for the blind. There is the Jaws program on computers. I own a machine that magnifies text up to sixty times. I have a handheld reading machine that photographs a page and reads it aloud to me. There are telephones designed especially for the blind and handicapped. At the Blind Center we were shown a small machine which identifies color. In San Diego, the Public Broadcasting Station provides a special reading service that can be heard on a special radio receiver. The Library of Congress provides tapes of magazines and books for the handicapped. And, of course, there is Braille. I am ashamed to say that I have postponed attending the San Diego Center for the Blind for years after the onset of my problem. Rule Seven: Take advantage of all the helps, mechanical and otherwise, offered to the blind. I know there are both guide dogs and training centers for the visually handicapped.

Rule Eight. I complain about many situations in the bigger world that are not tailored for those who are visually handicapped. It is easy to sit around and gripe or to suffer in silence. It is incumbent on every citizen that he or she speaks up for not only his or her own rights, but for the rights of others in similar circumstances to one's own. Rule Eight: The visually impaired person should join a lobbying group like the San Diego Council for the Blind to let those in authority know how society can help the living situation for all handicapped people. Of course, there are other avenues of protest, like letters to the editor, emails to Congress persons, and participation in political party groups.

Rule Nine. There is a temptation for the blind to become inactive, since certain kinds of activity are proscribed. It is easy for anyone, blind or not, to become careless about the health and usefulness of the body. Rule Nine: The blind person must take charge of her own health by exercise, diet, and avoidance of anything that militates against physical health. I suggest swimming and an exercise bicycle, yet I know visually handicapped people who play ball, participate in golf matches, surf, fish, and even run. Good general health cannot help having a positive affect on one's sight.

Rule Ten. I know that certain activities lie beyond a blind person's capabilities. I know also that in American society, once one has reached the age of seventy, he or she is excluded from opportunities of work and service. Rule Ten: The blind person, like any other person, must have goals for which he or she strives. Perhaps the goal is self improvement like becoming a better swimmer or piano player. Perhaps the goal is to develop some hobby like carpentry or gardening or stamp collection. Perhaps the goal is to find avenues of service like visiting sick people in a nursing home. To have no goals is to die before one's time.

With these rules, the croquet game becomes regularized. The hedgehogs become wooden balls, the arches become wire frames, and the mallets are made of solid wood and decorated with interesting colors. Even Alice, should she become blind, could play by these rules, and, above in the sky, the Cheshire cat would be always grinning approval.

CHAPTER NINE:

Mirror, Mirror on the Wall

Blind people, like everyone else, live in society, and their deeds and identities are shaped by that society. Robert Burns comments on how people are viewed by society in his poem "To a Louse" as he sees a louse climbing up the feather on a ladies hat as she sits proudly in church. The lady, tossing her head in pride with her fancy headgear, needs to be aware of how she is coming across to other people as they see the louse climbing up her hat's decoration. He writes:

> O wad some Power the giftie gie us
> To see oursels as ithers see us!
> It wad frae monie a blunder free us
> An foolish notion:
> What airs in dress an gait wad lea'es us,
> An ev'n devotion!

Like every positive thing, an awareness of what other people think of you can pose dangers. Such dangers are particularly present for the blind, especially those who become blind when they are young. Aware of the negative stereotypes that society possesses of blind people, many young blind people try to be acceptable to society by denying their blindness. The problem is that it is not easy to be hidden. What most of the blind come to realize later is that what they should reject is not their blindness, but society's stereotypes of blindness.

By reading the works written by the blind, we can discover the outlines of this problem. As a literature teacher, I should know that I might find out more about mankind in literature than in talking to my acquaintances. In good literature, the trivia and the disguises fall, and the true nature of the person and the condition are likely to appear. So if I want to know about how others cope with blindness, I should travel to autobiographies, to biographies, to memoirs, to fiction, to poetry, and to cinema to discover what one current blind writer has called, "The Planet of the Blind." From reading some of these books, one discovers just how damaging the attempts of the blind to disguise their blindness can be.

Georgina Kleege in *Sight Unseen* is very critical about how the blind appear in the mass media, especially in cinema. Since I cannot really see movies and Kleege is able at least partially to do so, I will refrain from analyzing movies on this score, since she's already reviewed movies to some extent. She sees the blind in the cinema being stereotyped as a poor lot. It is easy to see how these cultural stereotypes can impact the blind and make them want to escape their blindness. When she sees a blind person portrayed in a movie being pictured so miserably and as foils to the sighted, she is tempted to leave the theater in protest. Unlike how she sees her own visual handicap, she believes that screen writers portray the blindness as being central to the characters so afflicted. She asserts that blindness is only one aspect of her total being.

On the other hand, the blind characters portrayed in the movies have their whole lives impacted negatively by their blindness. Usually the blind are portrayed as unemployed, or having jobs in careers usually associated with the blind like musical performance or the caning of chairs. An exception of this she sees in *Sneakers*, where the blind person is a sort of detective. His detective ability, however, is stereotypical since he possesses extrasensory perception. She sees the blind character, never the protagonist, taking the role usually assigned to women: fascinating objects of scrutiny. She sees the blind portrayed as either asexual or oversexed, as in *Proof.* The movies present blind men as having a fatal flaw in that they cannot view and appreciate the beauty of women. In Alfred Hitchcock's *The Paradine Case*, the murdered blind man is seen as flawed for this reason. Blind women are portrayed even more pathetically as being creatures of desperate need. In *Jennifer 8*, Helena is saved from a murderer only by sighted people who surround her, and in *Wait Until Dark*, where Audrey Hepburn plays a helpless blind woman, the blind woman shows considerable skill only to end up cowering behind the refrigerator door and being rescued by a sighted man.

Kleege does not cast quite such a devastating glance at the books in which the blind appear. She starts describing how Oedipus blinds himself as the most cruel means to expiate the crime of the sexual violation of his own mother. Kleege describes at length the situation of Rochester in the novel *Jane Eyre*. Rochester's blindness is punishment for allowing himself to be attracted to Jane while his mad wife still lives in the attic. Fortunately his punishment is remitted after three years, and sight is restored to him, apparently by divine intervention. God is gracious. Kleege omits Elizabeth Barrett Browning's Romney, the social reformer whom Aurora Leigh rejects until his blindness puts him on equal footing with herself, humbling his masculine arrogance.

In her excellent memoir, Kleege seems to attack books written by blind authors as being too formulaic and somehow too self absorbed. The pattern begins to seem monotonous; however, short story critics usually describe the structure of the short story as problem plus resolution. Perhaps this structure is inevitable in a book that openly presents itself as a book written by a visually handicapped person. Should a book written by such a person simply list and present all the problems of being blind? I'm not sure that such a work would hold much interest for the reader. In any case, these books written by the blind are anything but formulaic in their honest and fresh portrayal of struggle and accomplishments. It is true that the formula is followed, in that they portray the onset of their blindness, its problems, and then efforts to cope with the condition. In her own book, Kleege roughly follows the formula and, like the books, she produces an excellent account of the world of blindness. I fail to see a radical difference between her autobiography and the others, all of which I see as fresh and enlightening.

Kleege herself sought to ignore her blindness by attending a regular school and avoiding the help she could have gotten from a blind instruction program. Her mother aided this attempt to minimalize her blindness by avoiding the word *blind* in describing her daughter. Her mother refers to her as having "neutral vision." Only later in life did Kleege learn to use Braille and a mobility cane. Although I cannot critique her description of the portrayal of the blind in cinema, I can comment on a number of books written about and by the blind.

Part I

When I was invited to give an address to the San Diego Center for the Blind, Kevin pretty much told me what I was to say, or at least the outline, and, of course, it was to describe how I overcame my handicap. To many people blindness is about the worst fate to befall one. Pity the blind. It is easy to elicit this pity. One summer I worked at a camp for handicapped youth. When we took the seventeen-year-old blind boy to church, and the elderly women of the church practically smothered the boy with money and sympathy, much to his chagrin.

Of course, some people like sympathy. At one school I taught, the young lady named Diana attracted like a magnet the sympathy of the entire college. Poor Diana. Pray for Diana. Diana's having a bad day. Diana has threatened to drop out of school, and truly Diana looked like a village that a cyclone that just passed through. Fortunately for my own psychic well being, I seem to repel sympathy. What would I have to do to get someone to weep over me?

One could expect, perhaps, that the initial reaction to blindness would be depression. Although there are some signs that people who become blind fight depression, the major problem to which the blind confess is the very denial of their blindness, not depression. I can certainly respond to this charge. Although I readily admitted to people that I had become legally blind, I fought against advertising the fact. For ten years, as I have cited elsewhere in this book, I refused to use a mobility cane. Not only did I wish to avoid attracting attention by using the mobility cane, but I hoped to avoid fitting into the stereotype of old age associated with people who use canes.

It is easy to understand why the blind shrink from being viewed so, since they adopt for themselves the stereotype of society that blindness is a result of some evil. In the gospels we read that upon encountering a blind man, Jesus was asked about the cause of the man's blindness. They chose two options to lay before him. First, that he had sinned, and second, that his parents had sinned. David Mehta, whose parents were Hindu, was the object of the following explanations for his blindness. His father maintained that he became blind because of a fever. His mother was sure that in a previous life he had done some horrible crime, like murder, and the punishment followed into his present life. She took him not only to psychics, but also to healers to find a remedy for his condition.

Accidents of birth, the excessive oxygen given to preemies at birth, and the natural deterioration caused by aging are usually named as the causes, not divine retribution or hard work. The poet Milton was blamed for the onset of his blindness as a result of the extensive reading and writing he did for the government under Oliver Cromwell. Eye specialists, however, are not ready to blame Milton's blindness on his exertions. In the sonnet "On His Blindness," Milton implies that Providence had denied him sight, complaining, "Doth God exact day labor, light denied." I am sure that the Royalists felt that he had the blindness coming to him for writing a defense of the execution of King Charles I.

Although most writers do not believe that blindness is some kind of curse, they do talk about the causes of their blindness. In no case do they attribute blindness to overwork by the eyes. In a novel *Katahdin*, the author Jason Trask describes the loss of vision by the protagonist as due to his staring into the sun while he was under the influence of drugs.

Upon hitting two snakes he saw copulating, Tiresias was changed into a woman by Hera. Ten years later, Tiresias witnessed the same phenomenon, whereupon Hera turned him back into a man. Later Zeus and Hera argued about which gender experienced the greatest pleasure in sexual act. Tiresias was consulted, since he had been both man and woman. Because Tiresias sided with Zeus, Hera struck him blind. The men of Sodom, according to the scriptures, were blinded as a punishment for seeking to rape the guests of Lot. Samson received from the Philistines blindness for his warlike depredations for their tribe. Had Samson not disobeyed God by revealing to Delilah the cause of his strengths, his locks would never had been shorn, and the Philistines never would have captured him and blinded him.

It is little wonder that blind children are tempted to disguise their blindness, since children are infamous for behaving like some animals that feel impelled to destroy that which is not normal or perfect. Stephen Kuusisto describes another problem that the visually handicapped face: students without eye problems choose to reject and tease visually handicapped students. Kuusisto records that sixth grade students ripped his clothes and beat him up, accusing him as being some kind of spy because he would sit by himself under a tree listening to sounds of nature. The most striking example of this is Rachael Scdoris. One of the great problems she faced was the relentless teasing and assaults she received in school. Here is another instance where some children can be absolutely thoughtless and cruel. She was teased because her glasses were thick. Boys would taunt her by holding up fingers and asking her how many she saw. She was called vial names and even fondled by boys. Girls were sometimes ever worse. They were quick to point out that her clothes did not match and were not stylish. In desperation she went to the principal and reported the language and the physical violence that she underwent. One parent made her son write a letter of apology. The parent of the second boy defensively questions why his son should be picked on because he does a little teasing. Interestingly enough the second boy never showed up at school again. These cases are not the only evidences of prejudice against the visual handicap that Scdoris faced. When she applied to the Iditarod Committee, they first turned her application down, claiming that she is asking for a special bending of the rules since she would require a visual helper.

We can say that the first obstacle the blind are challenged to overcome is the acceptance of their lot. The challenge is to admit that they are to some degree blind, and that, therefore, they will need to change the way they live and their appearance to others in society. The authors I read reported that they had attempted to deny their state rather than to accept their lot with equanimity.

The most extreme case of denial is illustrated by Kuusisto in *Eavesdropping* and *Planet of the Blind*. Only when he was an adult did he agree to use a mobility cane, like Kleege. Until that time he would attempt to hide his blindness by appearing normal. Not only did Kuusisto face problems with walking around campus and finding classrooms, but he was overwhelmed by his lack of ability to read the assignments and write papers. He, therefore, dropped out of his university training, in spite of the fact that he was informed that there was help for him both in navigating the campus and in studying. He appears to have been too proud and stupid to ask for that help.

Denying his visual handicap, Ryan Knighton, author of *Cockeyed*, insisted on borrowing his father's car, which ended up being stranded on a rock field. He did not let his father know that he turned into this rock field thinking it was a driveway, since he is visually handicapped. Then there was the time he sped across the four-lane highway without the benefit of a traffic light and sat while he contemplated the disaster that he could have caused. Another erroneous turn landed him in a ditch from which a tow truck had to extract the car. I believe that Knighton's avoidance of the fact of his blindness was much more severe than mine. He made himself miserable trying to pretend he was sighted, even teaching classes in Korea without letting the students know that he couldn't see well. He would venture forth onto the street, relying either on his girlfriend's direction or on his other senses. There is another great truth in the story. Knighton was consumed by his blindness. It colored negatively all of his life. He warns that blindness can fixate one's attention on oneself and one's own problems. In fact it may fixate one's attention not only on oneself, but on one's handicap. Hiding one's blindness can be a strategy that only complicates one's life. Throughout the first half of the book, this theme is elaborated on by his description of dozens of situations that describe this strategy.

Without any foreshadowing, Knighton writes about getting a phone call that changed his whole orientation to life and his handicap. His father calls and breaks the news that his younger brother, age twenty one, has died of a drug overdose, whether by accident or suicide. Suddenly and dramatically, Knighton assumes the role of comforting his remaining family members and arranging all of the details occasioned by his brother's death, including going through his brother's phone book, notifying all of the people therein about the tragedy. In the middle of all this description of the trauma, Knighton makes a simple but profound observation, namely that blindness, or any other circumstance, is only part of a person's life. One should not let oneself be defined by one's handicap. Along with that observation, Knighton comments that while the deaf form some sort of community because they rely on communication with each other, the blind form no such community. One cannot rely on other blind people. Each blind person is, therefore, an island. Because of the differences in the age of the blind, the degrees of blindness, and the diseases that cause blindness, the blind tend to be isolated.

Sally Hobart Alexander, faced with macular degeneration and detached retina as an adult, resisted becoming identified as a blind person. She attempted to continue teaching and continuing her relationship with her fiancé as if nothing had changed. Finally she moved from California back to her parent's home in Pennsylvania and agreed to go to the Center for the Blind there. The first days at the blind school were especially traumatic, since she was forced to confront her blindness. She felt that she would have no friends and no fun. She was ordered about by one of the supervisors like a robot. Losing her job, her relationship with her fiancé, and her independence all were difficult situations to accept.

John Howard Griffin, writer of two novels, journalist, and famous for his book on race relations, *Black Like Me*, was blinded by an impact of a bomb while he was on duty in the South Pacific. He became more concerned about escaping the Pacific after three and a half years of the war and being detained in a military hospital than he was about the state of his eyes. So eager was he to receive his discharge from the Army that he denied any wounds occasioned by the war. He was able to pass by the medical team that was examining him before his discharge in his eagerness to go back to civilian life. Certainly he could have gotten much help from the government because of a combat-related disability had he been more open. Reality hit him when he was informed that he could no longer continue with his medical studies because of his visual handicap. At least he accepted that judgment and turned his attention to music rather than medicine.

Avoiding the appearance of being blind is especially hazardous for one's physical well being. It is obvious that blindness presents a physical danger to people. Just walking about poses the risk of falling, bumping into something, or handling something that is dangerous, like fire. When a blind person moves round the town or city, she runs the risk of traffic or lamp posts or pits.

Both Ved Mehta and Tom Sullivan were so successful in coping when they were young with their blindness that they were not prepared for the impact of blindness on their later life. Mehta's physician father insisted that he not be confined to the house as his mother wished. Instead he joined a neighborhood gang of boys and got into all sorts of hazardous activity. In fact he would climb into places where his blindness shielded him from the danger he was in. Later in life he poses danger to himself by almost falling into a garbage elevator on Lexington Avenue in New York City. More seriously though, his refusal to talk about his blind condition with the four women he loved helped to drive each of them from him into the arms of a sighted person. Only with the help of a psychiatrist was he able to confront fully the impact his blindness had on his psyche.

Because his father insisted on his son's behaving as if he were sighted, Sullivan participated in all the activities of the neighborhood boys. His father urged him to engage in a boxing match and purchased a horse for him to ride. Sullivan never confronted his blindness totally until he found himself in a dormitory complex with other Harvard students and heard them talk resentfully about having to live with a handicapped person. His loneliness at Harvard led him to invite a woman he met on the bus to dinner in his rooms. When she failed to show up to the catered meal he had arranged, he left all the food uneaten.

Griffin describes an incident that illustrates the frustrations of moving about a room. Failing to mention to the manager of the hotel that he was blind and needed detailed help to get around the room, Griffin was frustrated when the hotel manager showed him to his room and quickly left, not pointing out to him where the bathroom was, or the telephone, or the bed. He, therefore, had to walk around the room with his hands on the wall and the floor, feeling out the environments of the place.

Bess Brennan had a special difficulty in accepting her blindness because it happened when a bully at school ran his sled into hers. She then had to realize that she was suddenly blind after being totally sighted. Her new disability came home to her with special force since she was a twin and found out that she could no longer go to the same school and pursue the same lifestyle as her twin. At first she refused to drop out of her regular school and go to the Perkins School for the Blind. Her uncle patiently persuaded both her and her mother to make the change to attend the blind school, where she could really be prepared to adjust to her handicap.

Perhaps more blame goes to the parents and other adults associated with the blind person than to himself or herself. In addition to their own personal denial of their handicap, the blind also endure the deliberate avoidance of the problem on the part of the adults. What is worse, they fail to provide for the handicapped child the special treatment that is available.

Kuusisto had parents and a grandmother who were at least middle class; he does not record their helping him to adjust to his blindness apart from seeking medical help. For a while in fact, he lived with his grandmother in isolation in the New Hampshire countryside. She seemed to have no friends, and he had none. It wasn't until much later in life that he was introduced to the mobility cane, Braille, and other helps for the blind. Had he gone to a boarding school for the blind, he might have gained a whole group of friends in his similar condition.

Knighton seems not to have had his eye trouble diagnosed in his growing up years. I am reminded of an inmate I met while I was a volunteer teacher at the Idaho

State Penitentiary. In the third grade, he was labeled mentally retarded because he could not read what was on the blackboard. No one bothered to discover that he needed glasses. This inmate said, "Had I been diagnosed as having eye problems, I would not have dropped out of school, and, in all likelihood, I would not find myself in this prison."

Part II

Oh with some power the gift to give us *not* to see ourselves as others see us. Sullivan was able to capitalize on his struggles with blindness to become an inspirational speaker on over 4,000 occasions. He tells his audiences that everyone has labels, not just the blind. One can be proud of his label if he accepts the challenge to make the most of his opportunities on a daily basis. He affirms that no one is ugly who does not accept the label. On the outside, the blind need to accept that they are blind, but reject the negative stereotypes that society forces on people. Only those who accept the stereotype that they are helpless and incapable of being effective doers need to be limited by prejudice.

One day at the San Diego Center for the Blind, in a small group, a blind lady confessed that when she was diagnosed with being blind, she retreated to her room and withdrew into herself. She was gradually learning that she had accepted the label of helplessness, and her first step in rejecting that label was to renew her study of the piano. All of the memoir writers that I have read have similarly eventually accepted their blindness, but not the stereotypes that go along with the condition. They refuse to see themselves as others see them. Against the stereotype that the blind are helpless creatures who creep around in their rooms and outside, accounts by the blind paint a different picture. The exploits of the blind prove that they are adventurous, capable, and daring. Kleege provides the most detailed account of her teaching success, describing how she manages to identify with the students and lecture to the students in a confident manner. She, of course, proves her excellence in verbal communication by the book she wrote. All of the accounts I read by the blind indicate that in spite of their handicap, they excelled in their academic work, and their writing is illustrative of their abilities. In fact other blind people like Kuusisto and Jacques Lusseyran achieved success in teaching as well.

Six of the most amazing accounts of blind ability can be found in works by Lusseyran, Sullivan, Mehta, Scdoris, along with James Holman and Fanny Crosby. Long before there were the modern helps for the blind, Holman set an enviable record of what the blind can accomplish. Holman's career in the British navy ended when he became totally blind. Rather than being content with retirement provided at Windsor Castle, Holman, against the rules of residency, made side trips from the castle to earn a medical degree at the University of Edinburgh. Before there were books in Braille, before there were tape recorders, before there were programs to assist blind students, Holman succeeded in earning an MD degree, even though he had to sit sometimes three times through classes. Lord Byron, a contemporary of Holman's, achieved fame by traveling first not through France and Germany, the usual path of the Grand Tour, but traveling rather to Spain, Albania, and Turkey, and writing about these adventures. Although inferior in literary ability, Holman far surpassed Byron in the extent of his journeys and in the number of books he wrote about his travels. Holman traveled well over 200,000 miles in his lifetime, venturing into Siberia and into Australia and New Zealand. While Byron prided himself on swimming the four miles of the Hellespont, Holman climbed Mt. Vesuvius. While Byron prided himself in being a good boxer, Holman became an expert horseman. He kept up his physical ability by running behind a carriage guided only by a rope which tied him to that carriage.

In the 19th century another writer proved her excellent ability and accomplishments. Crosby wrote over 8,000 hymns; at times she composed eight at the same time. Because many of her hymns appeared in hymnals, she often had to use pseudonyms, since the publishers rejected having too many hymns from one writer. Crosby achieved fame by writing secular poetry both about nature and patriotism, and she also composed lyrics for secular songs. In addition to teaching at a school for the blind in New York City, she became an advocate for the blind, receiving a warm reception in Congress. Her blindness did not keep her from meeting and recognizing many prominent lawmakers. She describes being in the presence of Jefferson Davis, later president of the Confederacy, sitting a few seats in front of her.

I can think of no more amazing accounts than that experience by Lusseyran during World War II. He was finishing his college studies in Paris when the Nazis overran France. At an early age, Lusseyran decided that it would be important to know the German language, perceiving that the conflict with Germany was imminent. Lusseyran would not stand by idly while his nation was under the occupation of the Nazis. Later in 1940 when Germany invaded France, he helped organize a resistance movement of university students and became editor of an underground resistance newspaper, active in writing, editing, and distributing the newspaper under the eyes of the enemy. Eventually he was betrayed and thrown into a prison in France. Later he was shipped to Buchenwald. Again he refused to remain passive; rather, he took on the role of piecing together what information he could find from rumors and a hidden radio receiver. From barracks to barracks in the prison, Lusseyran traveled to inform the prisoners of events taking place in the outside world. Thus, fellow prisoners recognized his importance as a contact with the outside world and a morale builder. Lusseyran records that one of the happiest moments of his life was provided by Russian and Czech prisoners who serenaded him on one of his visits.

After his early childhood of vigorous activity, Sullivan attended the Perkins School in Boston, where he became a champion wrestler as well as a brilliant student. Later at Harvard, he joined the rowing team and began his career as a performer at night clubs. As indicated earlier, he became a motivational speaker around the country.

After attending Pomona College, Mehta achieved excellence as a writer. In addition to being on the staff of the *New Yorker*, he wrote a number of books, especially on the nature of India in the modern world.

Scdoris, Holman, and Sullivan tout their physical abilities as high school students. Scdoris went out for track, ignoring the unexpected obstacles that sometimes appeared in the paths she was running. Early on too, she became a partner in her father's dog sledding adventures. It was not until she was eleven that she persuaded her father to let her run the dogs by herself. The track she ran was short, and he was watching; nevertheless, her act was a bold one. Guided by her dream of running the Iditarod, Scdoris learned to manage the breeding and care of the dogs and participate in ever larger sled races in the continental United States, such as the Race to the Sky and the Beargrease Marathon. Having proved herself as a skillful racer, she next had to fight for acceptance into the Iditarod race. The committee that ran the Iditarod was reluctant to accept a young blind girl to run this thousand mile race of endurance. Rather than pleading the disability act and exposing the prejudice of the

Iditarod board, she and her father managed finally to win the acceptance of the board. Although she was led by a dog team ahead of her, the leader of which communicated the peculiarities of the trail to her, she was required to be the sole racer on the sled and the sole caretaker on the trail with her dogs. The story of the 1,200-mile race is replete with dangers and crisis that challenged her unshakable determination to finish the race. Only when her dogs came down with an illness was she persuaded to drop out of the race. Later she returned to the race, this time completing it successfully.

Part III

Oh with some power the gift to give us *not* to see just ourselves as others see us, but to be able to see more than others see. Kleege mentions the bad associations that come with the term *blind*. So we have blind faith, blind prejudice, blind justice, the blind leading the blind, blind spot, turn a blind eye, blind as a bat, blindsided, blind chance, and blind rage. Since we live in a sighted world and so much of our learning comes from our eyesight, it is an easy assumption to make that the blind are somewhat ignorant, cut off from knowledge. However, so bountiful is the world in which we live. So limited are we in exploring its resources, and so marvelous is human ability and spirit that no one, sighted or blind, has begun to exhaust the possibilities of life. The old saying reminds us that it is an ill wind that fails to blow good to someone, and that every cloud has a silver lining. The pious say that God closes some doors in order to open others.

Unlike most of the media on which Kleege comments, she recognizes in "Cathedral" by Raymond Carver a wonderful exception. In the story, a man resents the oncoming visit of a blind man. To his surprise, the blind man breaks all the stereotypes that host had held, teaching him really to see the cathedral for the first time. From Tiresias onward, blind people have maintained that they have special insight in spite of literal sight. Others often view them, too, as possessing this religious insight. Far from responding to their handicap as Job's wife did ("Curse God and die"), they often seem to be in tune with the natural world and the supernatural.

One might suspect that with the loss of sight, the other senses become more acute and that the blind find enjoyment enhanced in using the other senses. No one describes the pleasures of sound better that does Kuusisto. Not only his loss of sight, but his isolation threw him into the world of sound. Even the daily sounds of nature and of human activity take on a kind of glory. Kuusisto would walk into the woods, sit under a tree, and identify the various bird songs. He noted the rustling of the wind and the gurgling of the stream. He could hear the faint movements of animals and birds as he sat quietly and listened. Kuusisto also enjoyed the sounds of human activity, like the guns of the Russian navy off the coast of Helsinki, the click of the train as it rushed along the tracks, the whir of passing automobiles, and the shouts of other children. Even while sleeping in his grandmother's attic, he would listen to the sounds of natural elements and the birds under the eaves, perhaps the reason for the title of his book *Eavesdropping*. He enjoyed visiting the circus with his father and listening to the roar of the lions and their rough breathing. Perhaps this sensitivity to the normal sounds around him prepared him for the delight of listening to music on the Victrola and later the radio. At a concert to which his father took him, he wept in ecstasy caused by the music that surrounded him. Once when he answered the telephone, Governor Rockefeller asked to speak to his father, who was a state official. Rockefeller then asked how the boy was doing. To the governor's delight, the boy then responded that he was enjoying Caruso. This acuteness of listening transferred itself to the listening of works of literature. Even though Kleege defends the quiet reading as opposed to the listening of books on tape or radio, Kuusisto listened to his father reading Mark Twain and books on tape with acuity and pleasure. Very few people enter the world of Milton's *Paradise Lost* as did Kuusisto.

Although Sullivan does not ascribe his love of music to his blindness, music played a dominant role in his life. In fact he ended up with a musical career rather than a career in counseling or business. His love of music got him in trouble with an intern teacher at the Perkins school since she accompanied him to various concerts, thus, bringing down the wrath of the school administration on her. Only coincidentally did he run into another Harvard student who was a piano player and began singing. The pair of them then began performing professionally, especially at night clubs in Boston and Cape Cod.

If Kuusisto emphasizes the glories of sound, Helen Keller, like John Keats, praises the tactile sense. She quotes Diderot, who says that while the eye is superficial, touch is the most profound. She illustrates her appreciation of touch in these beautiful words: "Hold out your hand to feel the luxury of the sunbeams, press the soft blossoms against your cheek, and finger their graces of form, their delicate mutability of shape, their pliancy and freshness. Expose your face to the aerial floods that sweep the heavens, 'inhale great draughts of space,' wonder, wonder at the winds unwearied activity."

Like Keats, Keller also praises the pleasures of imagination. Keats wrote "Heard melodies are sweet, but those unheard are sweeter; therefore, ye soft pipes, play on." Keller writes, "I reason that blindness and deafness need not pervert the inner order of the intellect." The classic example of this truth is, of course, that wondrous creation of the mind written by the blind Milton, *Paradise Lost*. Wordsworth, on looking out of his college window, viewed the face on the statue of John Newton and saw it as an index to "a mind forever voyaging through strange seas of thought, alone."

The blind have sometimes been viewed as possessing powers of seeing the spiritual world better than the sighted. The sighted Emily Dickenson wrote of this power of imaginative insight in her poem as follows:

> I never saw a moor,
> I never saw the sea;
> Yet know I how the heather looks,
> And what a wave must be.
> I never spoke with God,
> Nor visited in heaven;
> Yet certain am I of the spot
> As if the chart were given.

Scdoris combines what limited physical vision she had with spiritual insight. Although she could not see much of the natural world, on the Iditarod she is able to view the Northern Lights and writes about her reaction to them. "As night descended the heavens opened and the stars in the Milky Way shone with such intensity I turned off my headlamp... Those dreams from my childhood [of running the Iditarod] had finally become reality. But even in my dreams I had never imagined a night like this... If this moment were to last forever, I would be comfortable in the hereafter. I would never tire of a night so grand and glorious... Soon the Northern Lights began to sweep back and forth like broad curtains. Lights winked on and off, stretched, swept, lingered, faded, and then returned with even more brillance. The sky was alive... I believed He [God] was putting on this amazing display strictly for my benefit, and I might have been the only person in the universe who saw it. Out there, on that treeless plain of snow and ice, I was alone with God and felt as close to Him as I have ever felt.""

It is not surprising that John M. Hull would try to come to terms with his blindness through his faith. His father was a Methodist preacher, and he himself became a teacher of religious education. In the words of the hymn, Hull would probably say, "I ask no dream, no prophet ecstasies, no sudden rending of the veil of clay, no angel visitant, no opening skies; but take the dimness of my soul away." Hull's five-year-old son asks his father many questions about the nature of his blindness and the process of his becoming blind. Upon finding out that there's nothing medically that can help his father, the boy asked why God couldn't heal him. Hull feels led to accept his blindness as a gift. It is the gift of weakness, not strength, and it is almost as if God pauses before Hull's blindness in the same way that Christ paused before the cross. As Hull accepts the broken bread in the communion service, he accepts his own brokenness. "I felt that I was in the very presence of God, that the giver of the gift had drawn near to me to inspect his handiwork. He had drawn near as one who hardly dares to look upon the result of his work. If I hardly dared to approach him, he hardly dared approach me. I knew that he is infinitely great, with a mysterious beauty which is beyond all my understanding. I felt that he had paused, for a moment, and that soon he must be about his own strange work in worlds beyond my imagining. He had, as it were, thrown his cloak of darkness around me from a distance, but had now drawn near to seek a kind of reassurance from me that everything was all right, that he had not misjudged the situation, that he did not have to stay. 'It's all right.' I was saying to him. 'There's no need to wait. Go on, you can go now; everything's fine.'"

The most striking account of spiritual insight I read was written by Lusseyran. Imprisoned in Buchenwald for editing a French underground newspaper, Lusseyran escaped the nihilism rampant among some prisoners who became bestial and almost demonic in their actions. Lusseyran not only faced the deprivation and horror of Buchenwald, but found it accompanied by his own severe handicap. At the lowest point of his stay, when he was shipped off to a warehouse for the sick, Lusseyran experienced the sustaining power of God to such an extent that he felt that he needed nothing else. In fact he concluded that sustaining power was all that a human being really did need. His words really cannot be paraphrased. Here are a few of them: "I could tell by the pain my body was causing me, twisting and turning in every direction like snakes that have been cut in pieces. Have I said that death was already there? If I have I was wrong. Sickness and pain, yes, but not death. Quite the opposite, life, and that was the unbelievable thing that had taken possession of me. I had never lived so fully before. Life had become a substance within me. It broke into my cage, pushed by a force a thousand times stronger than I. It was certainly not made of flesh and blood, not even of ideas. It came toward me like a shimmering wave, like the caress of light… There were names which I mumbled from the depths of my astonishment. No doubt my lips did not speak them, but they had their own song: 'Providence, the Guardian Angel, Jesus Christ, God' …It is true I was quite unable to help myself. All of us are incapable of helping ourselves."

We often hear the question, "Where was God in the Nazi concentration camps?" One often hears the question, "Where was God in Auschwitz?" One might ask a similar question, "Where was God in Buchenwald?" Ask Lusseyran.

Since I have been paraphrasing for Burns' poem, I will mangle it again with these lines: Oh would some power give to the sighted, a view of the blind, as not benighted.

Chapter Ten:

Yes, We Can

Several times I have had the opportunity of speaking to graduation ceremonies at the San Diego Center for the Blind. It is one thing to write about blindness in the privacy of one's office; it is another thing to face the blind and partially blind in person. I knew that I was expected to give the audience of the blind and guests of the blind an uplifting speech. I certainly did not have to be forced to do so. For one thing I was at an institution, the very premise of which is that the blind can live meaningfully and successfully. For another thing, I believe in that philosophy myself and felt permission to testify that I myself have found life after blindness to be meaningful and enjoyable. I challenged my audience, as I had already challenged myself, to cope with life in spite of the handicap of limited vision.

I chose to divide the challenge of living life meaningfully into three categories. First, I stated that one can improve one's self physically, handicap or no handicap. Since visually-handicap people possess twenty-four hours a day like anyone else, there is usually no reason not to devote one hour of that quotient to the maintenance of good health. My own preference is for swimming, but others golf, play a modified form of baseball, softball, and walk. Even sedentary people can lift weights and perform calisthenics. In fact every morning at the Blind Center, everyone goes through a regimen of exercise. It is common knowledge that physical conditioning contributes not only to physical health, but emotional health.

Second, we handicap people have every opportunity to keep our minds stimulated and grow in knowledge and wisdom. The Library of Congress provides talking books free of charge to handicap people. No postage or late fees are required to receive these tapes. The Library of Congress also provides magazines on tape. A number of channels on television, especially Public Broadcasting System ("PBS"), provide cutting-edge information. PBS radio crowds the day with informational programs. In some places like San Diego, PBS also provides twenty-four-hour readings for the visually handicapped. Universities often provide access to classes for seniors, *gratis*. Libraries conduct book clubs and lectures. Books in Braille are available in libraries. The list goes on. If one, no matter how educated, stops learning new material, the mind stagnates and even regresses.

Third, there is no handicap that will keep one from reaching out to other people to lift their spirits by encouraging them and setting an example of meeting life with a smile. I remind them that Clay Potter, who was a student at the school, would learn everyone's name in the group. I could see him laughing and trying on homemade hats. I saw him move to the side of a woman in a wheelchair who he was told was having a bad day. I learned that, on discovering a hundred-year-old student had missed several sessions, he and another visually handicapped person went to visit the man and prayed with him. I recall one woman mentioning how lonely the coming Christmas holiday would be for her and asking if anyone would call her on that day. Six people quickly promised to call her and wrote down her telephone number. I ended this comment by quoting the sentiment that if you cheer someone else up, it is impossible that some of that cheer will not reflect on yourself.

Third, I challenged the assemblage to develop skills and abilities that might make them useful and give them a sense of accomplishment. I mentioned that I had still taught after becoming blind and that I was able to write a number of books. I mentioned Mary, who wrote poetry that was surprisingly good. It was handy that the blind David Paterson had become governor of New York State. I proceeded to mention the accomplishments of those already mentioned in preceding chapters. Finally, I stated that there is always a challenge to develop the human spirit and character. Is life not often more about what we become rather than what we do? I challenged them to remember people in their own lives whose greatness of spirit had enlightened their own lives. I talked about my Aunt Wilma, whose radiance of spirit spread to everyone around her. I mentioned a Mr. Harold Tyner, a retired man whose kindliness and dignity made a great impression on me as a boy.

I closed the talk by referring to the incident that I have already described, the occasion when the lady who had become mute through some trauma shouted out at a rally in Downtown San Diego, "Yes," and thus broke her silence forever. I chose to expand that one exclamatory word to a phrase, "Yes, we can!" I recap my talk by saying, "Yes, we can be physically fit. Yes, we can grow intellectually. Yes, we can reach out to other people, making friends and trying to help them. Yes, we can work on becoming the people we ought to be and what we are called to be." As I ended the talk, I asserted, "Yes, we can" three times. After the third "Yes, we can," the entire school stood and applauded. They let me know that they had accepted the challenge. Yes, we can.

About the Author

Art Seamans was reared in Upstate New York. He attended Eastern Nazarene College, Boston University, and the University of Maryland, where he received his PhD in English Language and Literature. He has taught at prep schools in the Northeast, Northwest Nazarene College, Mount Vernon Nazarene College, and Point Loma Nazarene University. At present, he is Emeritus Professor of Literature at that institution. He presently resides in San Diego, where he enjoys swimming, reading, writing, and occasionally teaching.